Lessons Learned Behind the Chair

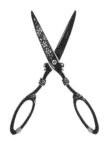

Kimberly McBee

Kimberly McBee

Copyright ©2019 Kimberly McBee – paperback.

Updated and Edited Second Edition. All rights reserved.

ISBN: 9781095586563
Imprint: Independently published

DEDICATION

To all the women and men who have sat in my chair.

CONTENTS

Acknowledgments

Introduction

Unrestrained Beauty College	1–64
Monday Morning Call to Adulthood	65–108
"Dazed & Confused" – The 80s	109–148
Next stage – A Doosy Day Job	149–166
Wild & Wondrous Wedding …and a Salon of Colorful People	165–264
Shenanigans & Surprises	265–286
Bumfuzzling — In the Chair & Out	287–324
Thank you!	323

ACKNOWLEDGMENTS

I sincerely acknowledge my husband, Mark McBee, for the enormous support he gave to me while I created this book—and for all the love he's shown over the years.

And to my children who I love more than life.

I wish to thank Nancy Beutler Abbey (NBA) and Judy Dippel for their encouragement and help.

I would also like to thank Jill for giving me the journal, so many years ago, that recorded the stories that I am sharing with you today.

My thanks to my many wonderful clients who have gone on this interesting journey with me—and for their loyalty, and for lots of laughs.

INTRODUCTION

In life, the most priceless written work exists in journals, or at least I think so! And we all know why—because within the often scribbled words and tattered pages is real life. Our tears and laughter, challenges and successes, dreams and reality, the bizarre and so-called normal, which includes the abnormal and unexpected that comes along in life—the truth!

My name is Kimberly McBee and I'm a hairstylist. I've kept the truth about the entertaining and crazy happenings of my profession to myself for many years, but I think it's time to share what I've written in my journal over the years. These are stories I couldn't begin to make up. What I've experienced highlights life—*Behind the Chair.*

In my chosen profession, I listen, hour-upon-hour, day-in and day-out! And so my journal writing began. I think most of my clients would agree that I sincerely care about them; the people who trust me with their hair! After all, they know a good cut and style rates up there with other really important things in our life—like kids, great coffee, and sex.

I'm revealing to you the stories that have come straight from my journal, and since I'm committed to being completely truthful, fact is, there are some people that are just easier to care about and appreciate than others.

For now—turn the pages and enjoy the interesting people and experiences of my life *behind the chair.* There's always lessons to learn… and the days are never dull!

Kimberly McBee

SIMPLY EGGPLANT

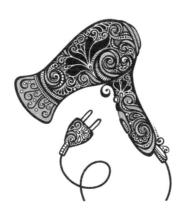

Writing down my stories all began on March 6, 2008, when a blank journal was given to me from a great client who I consider a friend—I'll call her Jill. *It was, and still is,* a colorful six-by-six inch, spiral bound, thick papered book with a beautiful Aubergine on the front—at least that is what the British call it. The image looks like a simple eggplant to me.

My name is Kimberly, but everyone calls me Kim, unless you are my mother who loves to call me Kimmy. And don't ask me why Kimberly was her favorite name to call out at me when she was mad, but I knew to watch out. It was Kimberly Dawn when she was really pissed. What is it with mothers who love to use their child's full names when upset or just plain red-in–the-face angry?

Anyway, back to this journal. Jill gave it to me as a gift, for the grand opening of my new salon. Yes, I'm a hairstylist. Not a beautician, as some people want to call the person behind the chair. I guess I could be called worse, but it's an old phrase that doesn't reflect what I do. Just like a flight attendant used to be called a stewardess. I know they like to be called that about as much as I like to be called a beautician. Not!

LESSON LEARNED
Stay up with the times on professional titles.

BONA FIDE BEAUTY COLLEGE

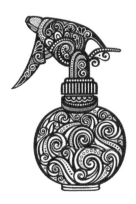

In September, 1985, I mourned the end of summer—the Willamette Valley kind of summers that are absolutely beautiful. They are not too hot in the rolling green hills of Oregon, where I have always lived.

That year, the leaves had not begun to fall, but I knew the rain was coming, and lazy days would soon be gone as I entered this new stage of my life.

I had graduated from high school in Pleasant Hill, Oregon, a small country town south of Eugene. Obviously, going to Beauty College was smaller yet, but even so, I was in for a big eye-opening experience of all kinds of people.

Sex, drugs and rollers!

Fortunately, for me at the time, my drink of choice was Mountain Dew, which I drank like it was going out of style.

I drove to school in my mom's Ford LTD red station wagon, because I had crashed my first car into a tree, a 1970 Plymouth Duster. But that's another story.

On my first day of Beauty College, we sat in wooden chairs with desks attached to them. The instructor showed us a video of people cutting hair and talking in a technical language that was English, but foreign to me. I put my head on my arm, on top of the desk, and woke to the instructor squirting me with a spray bottle full of water. If that was not bad enough, I had drooled all over the desktop. Everyone knew my name on the first day. Lucky me!

Thirteen was our class lucky number. I, along with eleven other women from all walks of life, all different ages, upbringings, and ethnic groups. And also one tall, well-built military guy who had just exited the service with an honorable discharge.

This type of man, in Beauty College, wasn't common then, so we wondered what *he* was doing there. We all know girls can be catty. That might be an understatement—since within any group of girls, there are those who are naive and others who can be downright mean. This group was no different.

Then there was Poor, Poor Sue, our instructor for roller setting and haircutting class. She must have been new to teaching. Her example wasn't the best. She stretched into her teenage daughter's jeans, trying to look younger. Her camel toe and dyed black-on-black hair was only outdone by her bright blue eye shadow and thick black eyeliner.

She stood teaching in front of student *number one,* who was fresh out of prison, a bowling-pin shaped woman in her early thirties. Next to her, was student *number two,* a curly haired, wide eyed, Jehovah Witness girl, newly out of high school. And then *number three,* Mr. Military Man with a twitch. I never had the nerve to ask if it was due to his military service, but he had quite a tic.

Numbers *four, five,* and *six* were cute, young, petite things that dressed alike, and looked like triplets since they even wore their hair alike. I thought of them as "the lovely three."

A bleached blonde, small spitfire describes student *number seven,* a nineteen-year-old girl, fresh out of a private Catholic high school. Numbers *eight* and *nine,* were two older women going through the change—menopause—including their slight midlife crisis. One, was going through a divorce and angry towards men. To myself, I called her, "angry divorcee." Her sidekick "southern drawl," was calm. She soon became the acting mother of the twelve others of us in class. She had "been there and done that." She was laid back, a good listener, and a lovely lady.

Short, I mean short-haired, know it all, happens to be *number ten.* She had done it, seen it, and pretty much could show you how to do it, whether you asked her to or not—know what I mean?

Number eleven was "the wild child." She was older than some, but younger than "southern drawl" and "angry divorcee."

Number twelve was a pretty young lady that came from money, and mommy owned a salon in town. I had the impression that she was forced to attend and follow in her mother's footsteps. Sadly, her head was too big for her body. *How does this happen?* It appeared that her body had stopped, while her head kept growing? I'll never know. I thought of her as "bobble head." I was afraid to bump into her, because her head might get off kilter and bobble around.

Lucky *number thirteen,* that was me! Eighteen years old, a five-foot-five blonde, quiet and sheltered, straight from a middle-class family in a small town. Little did I know that I was starting in a career that would open my eyes to the best and worst of people, and that it would be the life work that I would love—lasting for decades to come.

LESSON LEARNED

The far-out experiences of Beauty College could not end soon enough!

Lessons Learned Behind the Chair

HAIR CUTTING CLASS

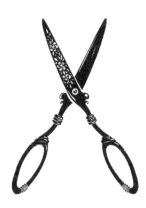

Poor Sue! She did not know how to teach one person at a time, let alone thirteen wise asses.

We were all issued our brand new doll head to start our haircutting class. They came to us in plastic bags—pretty scary looking. The doll's head was a regular human sized head, which was stuck on a pedestal that was clamped to the table.

The dolls had real human hair. The hair came from other countries where they grow their hair and cut it for money—sold for students to practice. The hair was treated for head lice, so it smelled. We cut them into tons of different cuts before finishing them off with a Mohawk or some funky style in the end.

One day, Miss Bowling Pin Shape, Straight-Out-Of-Prison, surprised us when she took her inner anger out on her doll—cutting the nose right off its' face.

When we started school, we were issued things,

kind of like the military does it. One pair of shears, commonly called scissors for you civilians. And we were given a hard suitcase that could kill someone if we were to swing it at them. It was black with huge silver snaps that kept it closed. Two doll heads to torture all through school; cut, bleach, perm, color. And if a head was lucky enough, it would not be one that was issued to "bowling pin shape" to have its' nose cut plum off!

One of our first lessons was to cut a straight line; a seemingly simple horizontal line on a strip of hair. At that, I thought I should pack my bags and head for the local community college and choose a different career. But finally, after practicing something I thought would be totally easy, I realized it was a challenge. And then, just when I thought, "I've got this," I was asked to cut a diagonal. I remember thinking, "Yeah, right!" But after 140,000 tries, I got it.

LESSON LEARNED
You can do *anything* you set your mind to…

NO RELIGION OR POLITICS

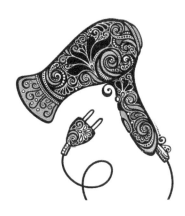

A few weeks into our classes, Poor Sue brought up religion. Granted, we were told in the first days of theory, not to start any conversation on religion or politics, *behind the chair*. But, Poor Sue went ahead and started something in our class that she regretted for the rest of her career as a beauty college instructor.

Poor Sue said something that started a conversation that lasted over a week about religion. We had a Catholic, a Jehovah Witness, Baptist, Christian, born again, and even an atheist.

Sue pretty much insulted everyone. Tears started when bleached white, spiky-haired Miss Know-It-All confronted Miss Wide Eyes, spouting, "You probably think all of us that are not your religion will go straight to HELL?" And Miss Wide Eyes, with her bouncy black curls, fought back tears and ran out of the classroom. She had never said a word about religion the whole week.

Needless to say, all the others then ganged up on Miss Know-It-All. The funny thing was, her statement wasn't really wrong, but it was the way she went about expressing it.

I'm not in favor of organized religion. I'm not saying I don't have my spiritual beliefs. I just think it's a personal choice people make and should not be judged. I love the idea of the Golden rule: treat people as you want to be treated.

Instead of the Golden Rule, I'll call it "Kim-isms." My mother taught, "If you don't have anything nice to say, don't say anything at all..." She never followed this rule mind you. :-)

I tend to say... if you don't have anything nice to say, shut your mouth! "Kim-isms."

Back at school, the name calling started. Throwing of rollers and hair clips, and combs and brushes got out-of-hand. I'm just glad we had not started with the hot tools!

LESSON LEARNED

Don't bring up religion or politics; it's really not worth the fight.

FAYE STEPPED IN

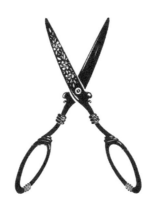

Faye stepped into the room, just as everyone was falling apart. The "Lucky Thirteen" group was in absolute chaos. Poor Sue, the instructor who had started the weeklong debate with the students, was crying and in the corner of the classroom. She had thick black eyeliner running down her face—combs and the hair clips that had been flying through the air, thrown at her, had accumulated at her feet.

I remember my eighteen-year-old self standing in disbelief, thinking... *what the hell just happened?*

Faye was the manager of the Beauty College. She was tall and slender, with smoker's skin and a rough smoker's voice. She sported a permed mullet! If you don't know what a mullet is—its business in the front and party in the back. It's a short cut over the ears in the front and long in the back.

Faye was old school HAIR. But she knew what she was talking about and knew how to teach, so all-in-all we got lucky. She became our teacher for the rest of our haircutting class.

Faye crawled up onto one of the classroom's wooden desks and started in. All I could think of while she was teaching the class, was to watch closely to see if she and the desk were going to tip and fall over at some point?

The desk should have not held her weight to the front side being very light; the desktop was not sturdy, but it held her without incident. But I think she had always lived on the edge. I believe she had been married several times, with cigarettes being her best friend.

She went on to enlighten us; she explained that really there were only four basic hair cutting techniques, and that by combining them stylist's achieved different haircuts. The basic bob: undercut the hair shorter, under the longer hair on top. The blunt cut: graduated, which you may know as a wedge, (hair cut at a 45 degree angle). The uniform layer: haircut the same length all over the head.

I looked at Faye, and her red hair which did not belong on a 50-year-old woman, let alone on any human head. I thought to myself, *she has three of those cuts just on her head alone!*

We discussed body structure and personality of the client, (guest) in our chair, hypothetically. We talked about face shapes, and I think at that moment in my life I learned more in the one-hour-and-a-half than I did in the rest of the theory classes.

In front of the class, Faye brought Miss Wild Child forward, demonstrating her long layered cut to us, which was perfect for her. She had a long face, and Faye pulled her hair up to look like the hair was cut short at her chin. We could immediately see that the length of hair emphasized her horsey face, which her wild, long blonde locks kept hidden.

Wild Child was not too concerned with the way the class was having an "aha moment" over the fact that she should never cut her hair short... *ever!*

Faye took us one by one and told us how she would change our lengths to enhance our looks, by wearing the correct cut for our face and body shape. Then she came to me—Lucky Number Thirteen. My hair was fine, and I knew for sure that during the summer I had been lying in the sun with as much lighting solution as possible, to make it transparent. (The sun penetrates your hair and if you put enough peroxide in before lying in the sun, it will burn holes completely through your hair.) She looked at my face and at my body. I almost felt as if I was being sized up. I felt uncomfortable. She then finally spoke." Well, mid-length hair is the best for someone with fine hair, not too layered and not all one length."

I think she just wanted me to go away—me and my damaged, thin hair. I envy women with beautiful locks. Some people just don't know how lucky they are. We always want what we do not have. If we have thick wavy hair, we want straight sleek hair. If we have straight, sleek hair, we want curly hair.

LESSON LEARNED
Work with what you've got!

And after all the chaos, what happened to Poor Sue? She got stuck with showing us roller placement. Today, that trade is almost all in the past. Who goes once a week to set their hair? Not too many. Washing hair once a week and having the stylist, or then called the "beautician," *do it up* is rare these days.

This reminds me of a lady who used to come to me once a week, but she would never pay with a check in full. Instead, she would write a check for about three-fourths of the bill and pay the rest in cash. She did not want her husband to know how much she was spending.

When going grocery shopping, she would write her a check for twenty dollars more to get the cash, so he would think the bill was higher. She would pocket the cash.

Funny how you can live in the same house with someone and even sleep in the same bed with them and really be lying or stealing from them, depending on how you look at it.

LESSON LEARNED
I would not stay married to a man like that.

PERSUASIVE INSTRUCTORS

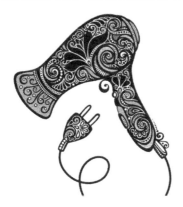

I enrolled in Beauty College thinking I was only going to focus on hair and make-up. I was talked into changing my plan by Mrs. John, the head of the college. She convinced me to take full phase, which means nails, cosmetology and hair. So I included nails in my *studies*.

The first day of nail class was a nightmare and really never got better. The fumes of the acrylic made me feel sick and dizzy in the small room with the doors shut.

Nobody knew what they were doing, except for one of the "pretty three." She had been applying nails from her bedroom on her girlfriends.

It was a weird way for us to try to learn, because our teacher didn't know much of anything either! I guess when you can't make it in a salon you go into teaching?

I somehow managed to put the prettiest set of hooves (horse's feet) on my friend, Miss Blonde Spit Fire. She was sporting around three pounds of acrylic on her nails, and they would have looked really great if she had been in a Budweiser commercial!

We bathed our feet in hot foamy water and worked on each others feet, and haphazardly manicured and polished each others toes. We studied all the nerves in the feet and hands, and all of the diseases and disorders of the skin. I hoped I never had to see them outside the book we studied. Who ever knew were over forty kinds of foot fungus?

LESSON LEARNED
Nails are a creative art, you either have it or you don't!

FAKE AND BAKE

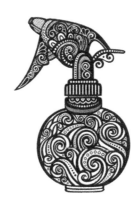

Off to cosmetology courses! The woman teaching this class was blonde, and she called her hair "frog fur" because it was a wispy, wafer thin denuded head of hair. In fact, she did not have much hair at all. What she did have was super fine. Still, she was an attractive woman.

She showed up in class always sporting fake eyelashes and self-tanner, applied generously. I thought of her as "fake and bake." Her skin was a little orange, but then in the eighties, it did not seem unnatural, since plenty of others had orange-tinted skin.

I give credit to Fake and Bake. She was good. She knew her stuff. She applied artificial lashes faster than a speeding bullet.

"Perfection," she would say, with a satisfied smile, after the second lash was applied.

We mudded up our faces, as we gave each other bad facials. We applied nasty make-up (age unknown) and wondered how many others had put their unclean hands into it.

Hair color class was my favorite. With no fear, (I was not afraid of this class) I would attack any challenge with color. I wanted to pick Fake and Bake's brain to learn more.

She had worked in salons for years, and had just started working at the college for added financial security, since her kids were going to the local university.

Formulating and learning the hair color wheel, was fascinating to me. I wanted to color everybody's hair that walked in the door.

I pulled their hair through a frosting cap with a crochet hook. Talk about pain. I often wondered who invented this torturous application.

Tin foil, who would have thought? Tin foil was just coming into fashion. Why? It was used to put natural looking highlights into hair, of course. Using a tail comb, I would repeatedly weave through a section of hair to put the foil under it, and then spread the creamy bleach onto the hair.

I love bleach. It's powerful! I once heard someone call it "the shark." Bleach will eat through things and kill pigment. It makes me feel like a rock star to turn someone blonde for the first time.

"What? You have never had highlights?" Famous last words: Poof your platinum!

LESSON LEARNED

Finding something you are good at can be a blast and a great job at the same time!

CLUELESS ABOUT CHEMISTRY CLASS

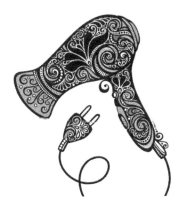

Who would have thought beauty school required a chemistry class? Not me! At least not when I was eighteen years old. It makes sense to me now, since chemistry is all about substances, and the investigation of their properties and the ways in which they interact, combine, and change. My hair color clients are probably glad I took this class.

The chemistry book that was given to us when starting this class was *thick*. We needed to learn chemistry due to mixing hair color. For example, hair dressers need to know the difference between acid and alkaline. I never would have thought of taking chemistry, but I found out I loved it.

Anatomy was another required class. This was *not* my favorite. It required memorizing lots of body parts and words that I could barely pronounce, let alone spell. Clearly, a career in a medical field was not my calling!

We all struggled and studied together. Since we had no way to know what would be on the test, to get the state license we knuckled down and studied until we completed all of it.

LESSON LEARNED

Most people do not realize Beauty College can be grueling.

Lessons Learned Behind the Chair

ON THE CUTTING ROOM FLOOR

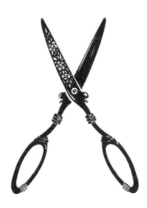

After about four to six weeks we were let loose on the floor of the beauty college, which means we got to cut hair on live, paying customers. Wow, these people walk into a beauty school and trust that the person standing behind the chair knows what they are doing. I call that "daring and courageous..."

My first patron was scheduled for 4:00 p.m. It was only 8:30 a.m. and I was already nervous. I had seen the woman's name, and I couldn't get her out of my mind. I wondered what she looked like, and I really hoped she was going to be nice. Of course, I didn't know anything except that her name was Silvia and that she always came into the beauty school to get her hair cut.

At 12:40 p.m., I was even more nervous. I wished she was coming sooner, because my heart was racing and my palms were sweating.

Suddenly, I hear on the intercom "Number fifty-six, to the front desk."

I stood still in my mandatory white lab jacket (paid for out of my own pocket, since it wasn't included in the cost of the tuition). However, each student received a stylist's number, and it was given free-of-charge!

My number was—you guessed it, number fifty-six. I had no idea why I was being called up front. I was up stairs minding my own business, drinking my fourth bottle of Mountain Dew, and trying to wait patiently until my customer came in at 4:00 p.m.

I walked down the stairs to the front desk. I reached the fake wood-panelled front desk, and the classmate working the desk said, "You have a haircut waiting in the waiting room."

I started to argue, telling her I didn't have a client until 4:00 p.m.

"Well," she said patiently, "There is a walk-in customer, and your number is up next."

What? Still in my brain I was thinking, *No, not until 4:00 p.m.* I took the ticket and somehow got my feet to walk forward into the waiting room.

There, I see a lady and a little boy who is about two years old. He looks like he really needs a haircut. I greeted her, and then told her I needed to set up. Like a zombie, I walked to the back as if I was not really in my body, finally reaching my station. I looked at the station, which was totally prepared and ready, since I had gotten it ready "for Silvia" at 9:00 a.m. that morning. Thinking, *I can do this,* I turned right back around and headed to the waiting room. I told the mother, "I am ready for him."

I grabbed a booster seat for the little man and a

miniature cape. This little man was not so happy. Apparently he did not think it was a superman cape!

I snapped it around his tiny little neck, after securing his blue Oshkosh bottom in the seat. His crying did not begin right away. He waited until I touched him with the comb. We both battled throughout the haircut. I think he won.

By some miracle, the haircut looked pretty good, but his mom and I were sweating and exhausted. She paid. I walked away with a sigh of relief, feeling like I needed a nap. The school collected the money for my first haircut. I knew the only money I would see as a student, is if the patron is kind and kicks me a dollar. This client was not that generous.

Four p.m. finally arrived. I walked to the waiting room as number fifty-six was called again. I felt steadier on my feet this time.

The room was crowded, and a half-dozen people stared at me as I entered the room. *Which one is Silvia?* I spotted one blonde bombshell, one teen that looked like he didn't want to be there, or that he liked to shower. There were two older women talking in a friendly, full-on conversation about what they could do with their hair to look younger.

One lady, in her mid-thirties, caught my eye with the biggest red mass of hair I had ever seen. And there also was a man that looked like he was stuck in the sixties with an outdated Beatles haircut.

I knew that my customer's name was Silvia, so my brain eliminated any male in the room.

"Silvia," I called out in a soft, shaking voice. The big red hair stands up and says,"That's me!"

I introduced myself, "Hi, my name is Kim." It's

nice to meet you, Silvia."

Thank God she could not read my mind, because I'm frantically thinking, *what in the hell am I going to do with this lady to undo her cave woman look?*

We reach my station. I'm sweating again, feeling the panic overtake me, as if I'm living a nightmare.

She sat down. I couldn't even put the cape on straight. I hoped that she didn't notice how nervous I was. She then said to me, "Relax man, I just want a haircut."

I let out a big sigh of relief. After her reassuring comment, I felt so much better.

I picked up my comb and scissors, and began to treat her like I had been doing this forever. Confidence! I'm *finally* feeling it, as I began to give her a layered hair style, shaping her wild red mane.

After I finished, I excused myself to search for Faye. I needed a sign-off from my instructor.

I walked past Poor Sue, and Fake and Bake, who were eating lunch. I finally found Faye, who was all the way in the back helping Mr. Military clean the brushes, so they would become hairless.

"Faye" I said, "I'm ready for you to critique my haircut." Faye followed me, and took one look at Big Red and picked up my comb and went through my cut. Then she looked at me with a straight face and said, "That's a nice haircut, Kim. Don't you think she should go shorter?"

I looked into the mirror at Big Red, and then the at the floor, realizing that she did not look much different from when she came in, except for the ends that I had taken off. So, once again, I started to cut through the thick, red strands. Faye told me to come get her when I had finished.

I took a second, more thorough look in the mirror at Big Red, and saw that she had nice features under all that hair. She was a natural beauty, and when I say natural, I mean natural—she wore no make up, Birkenstocks and hemp clothing.

I decided to create a fresh look for Big Red, and give her an unveiling. When I was all done, I renamed her "Sweet Silvia." She tipped me a dollar, all in quarters. She was my first experience of being paid for my work.

Then I searched for Faye again, for twenty minutes this time. I finally found her in her office doing paperwork.

Faye thought I had a new patron in the chair. She was very complimentary of the style and cut that I had given my big spender. Looking up at the clock, I was shocked to see that school had ended an hour before. This patient woman had been in my chair for three hours. She had earned her name, "Sweet Sylvia."

LESSON LEARNED

Patience is a virtue—especially in a beauty college patron!

Lessons Learned Behind the Chair

MODELS BEWARE

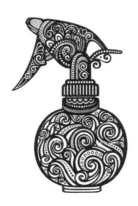

In color class, we were asked to bring in live models to practice our skills—ready or not! In return, the volunteer model gets a free color or highlights, and we got to practice.

So... I was really excited to offer someone my wonderful hair color service. My younger sister had a friend whose sister was pregnant at the time. I felt she might be a good candidate to be a model, because I don't think she had done anything quite like it before.

Her name was Jane, and she was a heavyset, pregnant woman. Even before conceiving a child, she was almost to the point of not fitting in the hydraulic styling chair. Jane was not just pregnant, she was ready to pop.

Jane happened to be a brunette, and through no fault of her own, was about to experience new hair color shock!

The instructor was a new hire! Yep, once again we had a new instructor. He was totally gung-ho on showing off new techniques. He was a tall, six-foot-two man, hair as blonde as snow, and feathered perfectly. The distinct smell of hair spray, to hold it stiffly in place, followed wherever he went, giving us strong whiffs as he walked by. He used so much, even when he stood in front of a fan, his hair would not move.

He wore blue jeans that fit so tight you could tell he was male. His "painted on" blue jeans made his junk embarrassingly visible. In a school full of young ladies, he definitely stood out. I was a little turned off. This was Beauty College, and considering it was full of young women in heat, they loved it. I was not at all impressed.

Jane showed up and as you can imagine, the stage is set. I had her take a seat and I stood behind the chair.

Six-Foot-Two began to direct me. "Kim, I'm going to show you a quick and easy way to highlight her hair."

He grabbed a vent brush and told me to mix bleach and 130 volume peroxide. (Normally you mix 20 volume with bleach—or at the most, maybe 30 or 40.) Overkill or not, I had no choice, but to go along with him since he was the instructor. After all, I was a mere student and new to color, right?

We took the bleach and smeared it on the plastic vent brush, and then applied it to Jane's healthy, virgin hair. In six minutes, her brown hair turned golden blonde, not just highlights, but her full head of hair. I was in shock. I just stared, speechless, at

Jane's ashen face in the reflection in the mirror. This was my first experience with a patron in pure panic mode! I hoped she wouldn't scream, or worse yet, faint!

I hated to even think it, but as Jane sat looking at her reflection in horror, it was time to start the bullshit. I conjured up phrases in my mind: *you look great as a blonde; this color emphasizes your eyes; what a great time in life to be blonde.* However, no words escaped my lips; I just stood there, speechless. Jane, big and pregnant, had come in for highlights, and now, sadly, she looked like a trailer trash blonde. What could I say to her? "Well, you will love it. I sure do!" *Not.*

"You are going to stand out in a crowd." *That's for sure!*

"Blondes have more fun." *Well, I thought, maybe not this blonde! :)*

The owner of the school walked in right as my panic over this struck an all time high. His name was Art, Art Waters. It was like some famous movie star walked in. It was the first time I had met him. Oh, what timing!

He walked over and saw what I was in the middle of, and his face said it all. His brows creased, his eyes got dark and angry. His face turned red as he set his jaw. He didn't have to say a thing. I told him exactly what Six-Foot-Two had told me to do.

I could see my own panic reflected back at me from the emotions in Art's face. His eyes showed his anger. Needless to say, that was Six-Foot-Two's first warning from Art. Undoubtedly, there would be many more to come.

I saw Jane months later, quite a while after the color episode that had turned her into a three-hundred pound Marilyn Monroe look-alike. Fortunately, she seemed to take it in stride—*she was still speaking to me*—and at least the outrageous concoction hadn't burned all of the hair from her head.

Jane was carrying her new baby girl, and she had two inches of dark grow out. I never, ever made that mistake again. A great learning experience, never to be forgotten! Thanks, Six-Foot-Two.

LESSON LEARNED
Blondes do have more fun!

LUNCH TIME REALITY SHOW

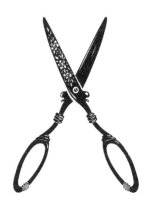

Lunch time was an experience in real life every day. Have you ever seen a movie taking place in a jail lunch cafeteria? Well, it was not all that bad, but it best describes the atmosphere and feel of the beauty school lunch room. The room was a just a break room, upstairs and had no windows. We sat at long formica tables. A pop machine stood in the corner, which offered a spot of color in the otherwise bland room.

    The machine was handy, because I drank good ol' Mountain Dew for breakfast, lunch, and often one more for the road after school. The machine sold pop for seventy-five cents. Getting tips in quarters worked great—like the first four quarters I got from Sweet Silvia.

    During lunch, I would sometimes go into one of the empty classrooms and crawl under the table for a nap. I seemed to need it since I got to school at

8:00 a.m. and left by 5:00 p.m.—like a *real* job. That's what they wanted students to think anyway. But the funny thing is, ever since starting real jobs; it's never been a straightforward 9:00 to 5:00. I've worked 9:00 to 9:00 lots—and even 9:00 to 11:00, but that's a worthwhile topic for later stories.

For now, I want to take you back to the jail house lunchroom. At that time, students were allowed to have a smoke. I didn't smoke then, and never have, but lots of stylists/students did. We all consumed the haze of smoke during lunch, so I might as well have smoked!

In this lunchroom, there was a tiny one-room bathroom with a small sink and one toilet, only separated from where we ate by a thin, almost pointless door. If we needed to relieve ourselves, and didn't feel like walking down stairs and using the public restroom, we could use this one. Not good though, because everyone knew if you were going "number one" or "two." Oh... and another way they knew— no fan! No question, I always used the public restroom downstairs,

The college was located in the middle of a small town—Springfield, Oregon. Fast food was near us on a couple of corners, and also a Chinese restaurant. If you wanted to get fancy for lunch, there was a bistro. I loved Bob's cheeseburgers, so often I went there for fast food.

Blonde Spit Fire, my buddy, would walk over there with me, since Bob's was basically in the back parking lot of the school. Blonde Spit Fire, or Fire Cracker as I often called her, had close set, pretty blue eyes and stood about four-foot nothing. She lived in an apartment in the same town as the college.

I still lived at home in the small town of Pleasant Hill, about a thirty minute drive out of town. I was intrigued with living on my own, but was too broke to do so. Spit Fire's parents supplied her enough money to go to school and live on her own. She had spending money, and did pretty much whatever she wanted. She was kind enough to take pity on me and buy me lunch once in a while.

One day, as we walked back from Bob's Burgers, there was a car parked in the alley. Smoke billowed out of the windows—*sweet smoke.*

I stared, and my mouth fell open when I saw three of my classmates smoking out of a pipe, and it was obviously not tobacco. They stepped out laughing. They were higher than a kite. A few feet more, and I saw another car in the alley, and Six-Foot-Two and Bobble Head were doing lines with the Pretty Three.

My eyes opened wider as I saw the mirror and white cocaine lines they were cutting neatly with a razor blade. They openly snuffed it up their nose with a short straw. I had seen marijuana before, but never white drugs. It was the real deal and a bit shocking to me that they were doing cocaine lines at all, much less at lunch. In my book, this wasn't lunch food!

As we rounded the corner a student who was not in our class, but had been in our school longer, (they call them seniors), got out of a brand new shiny truck. She reminded me of a pixie, energetic, small and petite.

"Dawn!" I asked, "Whose truck?" I didn't think it could possibly be hers, since she had told me she was on state assistance.

"Mine," she said with a smile ear-to-ear. I started to wonder if she would have the truck repossessed next month or a few months from now. Clearly she would not be able to withstand a brand spanking new truck payment. Then I thought... *Who knows? Maybe she is stripping on the side.*

And what about me? Well, as I walked by her, I just smiled, trying to be cool, as I popped the last French fry in my mouth. Then I cringed a bit when I spotted my mother's bright red LTD station wagon that I drove—it was as big as a boat. *Not cool!* However, it did have one unique feature. It was equipped with an electronic horn that played seventeen different tunes. (My sarcasm at its best—*get this mockery and you get me.*)

LESSON LEARNED

I quickly figured out I was not as naughty and worldly as I thought I was—and that lunch time definitely was not for wimps!

WANT TO DANCE?

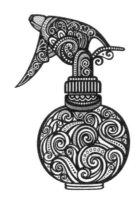

In the evening, after Beauty School and after work, Jenny, my friend from high school and I liked to go dancing.

Jenny was not the brightest match in the box, but she was a pretty good friend, and I enjoyed doing stuff with her. She never drove, so I did all the driving. We were nineteen, and loved to go out dancing at the "under 21" clubs around town. We even drove up to some of the dance clubs in our state's capital, an hour away. That was a big deal then.

One Friday evening, after I finished at school, Jenny and I decided we wanted to go shake what our mama gave us, so we headed to downtown Eugene and went to a place called "Players." I looked like a wreck, so I wasn't too excited about showing my face. I was glad Players was dark. We arrived and showed our ID's to prove we were over eighteen. The music was loud and the lights were shining on the mirrored ball going around and around.

Jenny got asked to dance right off. To be frank, Jenny was blessed in the boob area, so the guy's always zeroed in. I laughed to myself, because she loved it.

After one song, I felt someone staring at me. I looked up, and on the staircase was a handsome, muscular, dark haired, dark skinned, blue-eyed guy watching me. He mouthed something to me, and I looked around, presuming he was probably talking to someone else.

He proceeded to come straight down the staircase and walk right over to me.

"Hey," he smiled, and I smiled back and said "Hi." I could feel the blush rise in my face, not meaning to show that I was self-conscious. He asked me to dance, and I said, "Sure."

He talked to me all the time we danced. "My name is Logan." he said. I'm twenty.

An older man! I thought.

I quickly replied, "That's cool," and told him my name. We danced and talked until the end of the night. Logan walked me and Jenny back to my car. At that time, I was driving my 1970 Plymouth. As we got in the car, he told me he would like to take me out sometime on a date. I agreed, and we exchanged phone numbers.

He then walked to his little red Toyota, a four-wheel drive truck and hopped in. I was so excited. Before this, I had only dated boys from highschool.

The first date with Logan, he took me to a well-known restaurant in town. We chatted comfortably like we had on the night we met. I told him I just had started Beauty College—and added—"I work in a fast-food restaurant that serves roast beef sandwiches—I hope I don't smell like one."

He reassured me that I didn't, and told me that he was a choker setter for a logging company. He shared that he had to get up early, and be on the log landing by sunrise.

WOW, I hate getting up early... I thought to myself.

Logan and I really hit it off, and after our first date we were officially boyfriend and girlfriend.

LESSON LEARNED
Sometimes you find what you are *not* looking for—and when you least expect it.

Kimberly McBee

A LIMO?

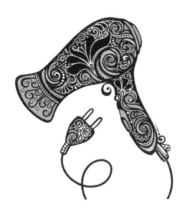

One day Logan showed up at the Springfield Beauty College in a black limo, after we had been dating for about three months.

I liked his look and personality, but I was not impressed with how he handled his finances. He had a responsible job as a choker setter (logger). It paid good money, but I never knew where he spent it. He got paid, and always by the third or fourth day after, he was broke. He lived with his sister and brother-in-law and slept on their couch, so I knew it was not going towards living expenses.

Well, here came one clue! One day, a limo drove up right in front of the windows and glass door of the school. All the girls were giddy and curious about who could be in it. Obviously, in Springfield, Oregon, we did not see limos on a regular basis.

Logan stepped out of the car as the driver held the door open for him. I was so surprised, but his long curly black hair was looking great that day. *First thing I noticed as a student of hair!*

Wearing a silky black, button down shirt and blue jeans, with new cowboy boots that he had bought for the occasion, he looked hot. All the girls in the college were yelling and screaming, "Who is that?"

My friend Mary said casually, "Oh, that's Kim's boyfriend." I had introduced Mary, a student in the class behind me, to him and to his best friend, and they had started dating.

I made my way to the front of the waiting area and saw the limo and blue-eyed Logan out front. The wind was blowing, and the dozen red roses he was gripping were taking a beating. All the girls were screeching for me to go out. I did, but was worried what might happen. I just had this awful feeling that he was going to do something really stupid and put me under a bunch of pressure.

I wanted to run out the back door, and jump in my mom's big red LTD station wagon to escape, but there stood Logan—there was no escape. He grinned a huge heart-melting smile when he saw me through the window, showing off his huge, perfect pearly whites.

I took a deep breath and stepped outside. I was wearing a white wrap around dress and it got caught up in the wind. It felt awkward; there certainly was nothing Marilyn Monroe romantic about the wind whipping at my dress.

"Hi," I said timidly, as he grabbed me around the waist and kissed me. "Want to go for a ride?"

I agreed.

By now all the girls were out on the sidewalk, whispering and envious as we got into the car. The driver gently shut the door behind us, then got into the driver's seat and started the engine.

Logan could not wait another minute. He took out an engagement ring and proposed, right then and there. I know this may sound romantic, but I felt pressured from such an extravagant display with the limo, and realizing everyone probably knew what was happening. I had the feeling he did it in this splashy fashion so I could not say no. After all, we had only dated a short while, and right then I did not know if I even cared enough to stay together, let alone get married to this young man.

Even so... I still said "Yes," and regretted it for months. We planned a twelve month engagement. It lasted nine. The breaking point came when we were at my mother's place and got into an argument over who knows what; I don't even remember. He ended up walking back to Springfield, where he lived with his sister, which if you drive, takes thirty minutes.

He didn't tell me he was going to leave; he just left when I wasn't right there. I looked for him, and then finally called his sister's home in Springfield. He answered. He was short on the phone and told me he had hitchhiked back to his sisters. He said he would talk to me later. He cut me off short, not caring about my feelings or anything I had to say.

Right then, even though we were still engaged, I decided not to put too much effort into calling or getting in contact with him. I decided to let him chase me.

Logan was mad because I had pictures of my

highschool boyfriend; prom pictures in an album. I thought it was childish and stupid that he could be mad at that. He showed how controlling he was, because he made me put my photo album of high school pictures in the fireplace, and before I could retrieve it, unknowingly, my mother lit the fire.

He never called or stopped by for three weeks. This just proved what I had known in my gut all along—he would not be the ideal husband. My decision was made.

A few days later, I went over to his sister's house and knocked on the door. His tiny little niece opened it with a huge smile. I asked to see Logan, and she opened the door wider where I could see him asleep on the couch. I walked in and woke him, and told him I was sorry this was not going to work out, and gave him back the engagement ring. I felt relief flood over me! I knew breaking the engagement was the best decision I had ever made in my life.

LESSON LEARNED

Never settle! Alway's pay close attention to your gut feeling if "this is right" or "this is wrong!"

MY BELATED FATHER

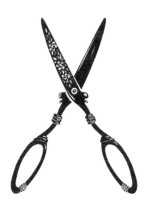

How would life have been different? This is a question I sometimes have asked myself over the years, because sadly, I never got to meet my biological father. His life was taken before I was born.

I have often wondered if he had lived, and if he had been able to love and guide me, would it have made important decisions easier, like the engagement and breakup with Logan.

Would my life be different?

My mother was pregnant with me when he was killed while on duty working for the Eugene Fire Department. At the time, my older sister was seven, and my brother was five.

It happened in October, 1966. My father was called in on his day off to help fight a horrific fire in downtown Eugene. A local car dealership and repair shop was on fire.

My father's life was taken that evening, and I

never got to meet or know this man. My whole life, I have only heard wonderful, almost super-hero things about him. Jack of all trades, smile from ear to ear, and could talk my grandmother out of anything.

I think I know the answer to my question—yes, my life would have been different, but in what ways? I'm not sure, but of one thing I can be sure—I am grateful to know that my father was a good and respected man.

LESSON LEARNED
Sometimes in life we are left to wonder—and we will never know.

TIME CLOCK

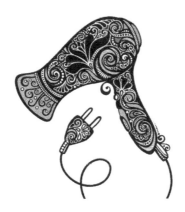

In Beauty School, we had to punch a time clock, once in the morning, at lunch, and again after coming back from lunch, and then yet again when we left for the day.

We needed a specific number of hours to graduate, plus we had to pass the "baby board test" (the practice test of the state board test we needed to get our state license), and several practical tests.

Plus, we were required to do a certain number of each service that is offered: so many haircuts, so many perms, so many pedicures, and more. I'm sure you get the idea.

The day I was going to perform one of my last perms needed to meet my quota, a lady was given to me named Daisy. No, she did not look like Donald's girlfriend and she was not dainty like a flower. She reminded me of an older Faye.

I took one look at her and thought...

CONDITIONER STAT! Then I positioned myself

behind the chair to start my consult, which we were taught to do with each patron. Standing in front of the mirror behind her and the chair, I was wearing my *not so white* lab jacket that had one pocket with a little hole in the bottom seam, and was slightly freckled all over with color spots.

I introduced myself and asked, "What can I do for you today?" She did not even make eye contact as she snapped back, "I'm here for a permanent."

I knew this was not going to be easy. I gently asked her, "Have you had a perm with us before?"

"Yes," she snapped at me again.

I left her to go look up her record card. As I read it, I saw that she had previously gotten the cheapest perm, and the smallest, tightest rods known to man had been used. I rolled my eyes at one of the girls at the front desk, as she gave me a sympathetic look. She had either heard the conversation or had had her own encounters with Sweet Daisy.

I walked back to my senior station in the front. And with confidence, I examined her record and asked her if she would like to try a more conditioning perm this time. I hit a nerve! Her response made it seem that I had said something really insulting. "OH, NO CONDITIONER! I want the perm that costs nine dollars and no cut—I cut it myself, and I know you will charge me more—*so no CONDITIONER!*" Daisy snapped angrily at me again.

I went on to explain to her how there was no way her hair would take the perm well without conditioner. I tried to make it clear that I could happily give her the same permanent she had had last time, but her hair needed a conditioning treatment first.

This time she practically yelled—
"NO CONDITIONER!"

I was stumped. I knew if I did what she was asking, I'd be in trouble. I simply could not wrap her hair in the dry condition that it was in—with her wonderful home-done haircut, which only added to her harried look. Pausing, I excused myself, and made a frantic walk/run for Faye.

As usual, Faye was once again doing paperwork back in the school's office. I told Faye my dilemma as my heart raced.

Faye opened a cabinet door and pulled out a piece of crisp white paper. The paper was a consent form for patrons to sign. It ended the need to try to convince her, because it stated that if she didn't follow our advice and we did what she asked, we were not responsible for the outcome.

I left the office and walked back to my station, feeling some relief as I walked through the waiting area, and on to the salon part of the building. With backups, I marched straight over to Stubborn Daisy. Faye followed right behind me for moral support.

We both arrived at the perming station about the same time. Daisy had a look of total impatience on her face. We thoroughly explained the paper she needed to sign—and why.

We both strongly encouraged that she take our advice and be more kind to her hair. She impatiently glared as we spoke to her. She was determined to get what she had last time, so she grabbed the pen from me and signed it with black ink aggression.

Faye signed it as well, and took the paper. She smiled slightly... "Have a nice day," and walked back to the office, leaving me there to do the bad deed.

I calmly draped Daisy with the normal routine, for her three-hour permanent wave. With a fresh crisp white towel around her neck, draped under a shampoo cape, and the velcro stuck firmly, I asked her nicely to please follow me. Truth be told, I wanted to keep walking right out the back door, *by myself*, and hop into my Big Red LTD station wagon and drive home to my mom.

She stood up from the chair, and made a satisfied "smirk and sniff" as if to say, *I got my way!*

I did the shampoo only. *No conditioner!* Seriously, there is good shampooing and bad. I have had someone use my head like a jack hammer when shampooing—and yes, I would call that bad. A good shampoo is delivered differently—and it is relaxing and soothing, and gives shivers up their spine.

I'm going to tell you a little secret if you are a stylist. You can keep clients by giving them a well-done shampoo. I, myself, have had great shampoo's that last longer than others and keep me thinking about it for days after. Almost as good as sex, but I won't take it quite that far. I can personally say, at times, there have been better shampoo bowl moments than bedtimes at some points in my life.

Now, back to Sweet Daisy. She followed me to the chair after I had given her a great shampoo experience. She sat up straight in the chair, more relaxed, almost seeming like another person. She still would not give me eye contact and that was okay. I was going to do as she asked and cross my fingers and hope that it turned out well for her.

I retrieved my basket full of tiny red and yellow perm rollers. These were the smallest know to women. The red were as small as a toothpicks and the yellow slightly larger. I had a box of papers to wrap around each section of hair that would surely curl into sheep's wool curls.

After about an hour of rolling, I was on the last section of hair. I told her I would be back in a jiffy. I had to go get the cheap jug permeant wave solution, which, of course, I didn't say out loud.

The problem with this was that all the students poured out of this jug and some of them did not put the cap back on tight. This caused the solution to weaken. I stared at it, hating to use it, but Daisy asked for this specifically—or should I say she demanded it?

Here goes nothing! Back at the chair, I grabbed a strand of cotton and and wrapped the cotton around the perimeter of her head, so that as I put the solution on each roller, it would not run down her face, neck or into her ears. I finished, and then placed a plastic bag over her head, making it snug to keep heat in... and off we went to the dryer chair. I now renamed her, Dazzling Daisy, hoping this would indeed be true in the end. I placed her under the hood dryer and asked if she would like a cup of coffee or a magazine. She grunted something incoherent at me, which I took as "No." I set my snazzy egg timer, stuck it into my pocket and walked away, knowing that I had twenty relaxing minutes *without* Dazzling Daisy.

With a deep breath, I headed upstairs to my jail house lunch room, straight for the sugar-laden pop machine. After twenty minutes, the timer went off. It was time to take a peek at her under the dryer. I could see the dryer was plenty hot, because Dazzling Daisy's face was hot pink.

I opened the dryer and she seemed startled, even though she saw me walk up and smile at her. I looked at the curl formation to check the wave pattern. Daisy looked like she was thoroughly cooked.

I kindly asked her to follow me back to the shampoo bowl, where I rinsed her with warm water. I then dried her head, still full of tiny little rollers, and then again, I took a snake-like shape of cotton and wrapped her curled head. She was looking tired, so I told her, "We are on the last stretch." She completely ignored me, acting like I had said nothing at all.

I put the neutralizer on the curlers in her hair, one at a time. Since patrons go from the very warm dryer to a warm-water rinse, I had learned to set the bottle of neutralizer in a bowl of hot water so people don't get the urge to pee when the cold splashes on their head. It seemed really mean to put the freezing cold neutralizer on them. I must admit that I did think about not heating it for Dazzling Daisy though.

I set my trusty egg timer for five minutes this time, and decided since Daisy was not much of a conversationalist I would clean up whatever I could to get things tidy. This kept me busy, since pleasant conversation was not an option.

The timer finally went off, and strangely enough, I was more than ready for this client experience to end. I began to take out all the hard work I had done, dropping the tiny rollers in the sink. Next, I rinsed the head of new curls in the shampoo bowl one last time. I sat her up and dried her full head with a white fluffy towel. We then walked back to the station so I could unveil the new Daisy, curls and all. Daisy took one look in the mirror and seemed pleased.

"Would you like me to set your hair today?" I asked.

Not surprising, she answered "No!" ...stating that she liked the wash and wear look." *Figures...* I think to myself.

I took the superwoman cape off, and removed the wet towel around her neck. She stood, and practically flew to the front desk to pay. I followed behind her with the ticket. Nine dollars is what is asked of her, and that is what she paid, not a penny more, no quarter tip, or not even a "Thanks, kid."

ONE WEEK LATER

Daisy suddenly barreled through the glass front door of the college. I saw her from my station where I was cutting a young woman's hair who had become one of my regulars. My veins ran cold. Daisy looked like a cotton frizz fest. I wanted to run and hide. I knew what was coming.

She yelled, *and not quietly,* at the front desk student of the day. "I want to talk to the manager!"

I'm sure everyone in the school could hear her. Daisy slammed her big orange purse on the counter. Her face was a nice shade of red, which made the frizzy afro on top of her head display a clown-like appearance.

Faye came out of the dispensary with not a

flicker of distress. I admired Faye's strength. "Yes Ms. Hill." Faye said with a smile.

"Just look at me!" Dazzling Daisy, AKA, Ms. Hill screeched. "I don't even have to tell you, just look at my hair!"

Faye gave her a firm look and got into the draw under the counter of the front desk and pulled out that wonderful piece of paper Ms. Hill had agreeably signed one week ago.

She stared at the paper, knowing there was no way to argue her way out of this. Faye calmly said, "You did not take our advice and this is the result. I'm sorry you chose to not follow the professional's advice, because if you had, you would not be in this predicament."

I stood a little taller, because that was the first time that I was called a professional!

LESSON LEARNED
Alway's do what is best for the clientl

Lessons Learned Behind the Chair

EYE-OPENING FIELD TRIP

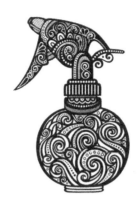

Lucky 13 got the opportunity to go on a field trip to salons around town. Blonde Spit Fire already had a job, due to her parents knowing the manager, and she was really excited to take us by to see where she was going to be working.

Her job would be in the local shopping mall, near the river. Blonde Spit Fire would be at the Montgomery Wards Salon, one of the bigger anchor stores in the mall.

The Pretty Three, hoped to work downtown. *Of course*, all three wanted to work together. They also had their eye on another salon that was also in the mall. It was a very chic salon. Many people with money went to this salon.

I knew that I never wanted to work in a salon where the stylists ane clients who went there had their noses stuck up in the air and thought they were better than the rest. I already knew that I wanted to be a hairstylist who cared about the people that would be sitting in my chair, and I needed to work somewhere that supported that philosophy.

The time came for our field trip, and off we went in five different cars, one after the other. I rode in Fake and Bakes car. She drove a nice town car.

We first went to visit the downtown salon. They had set aside an hour for our tour and questions. The man who greeted us was kind to take time out of his busy schedule.

Standing in front of us, he didn't mix words when he said, "You have picked the wrong profession. You will work long hours, your feet will hurt and your back will ache." He went on and on…

You know what? He was so right about the logistics of it. But he was not right about it being the wrong profession, because after over thirty years, I still look forward to stepping behind the chair every work day. He enjoyed hearing himself deliver his long drawn out speech, even if we didn't. We all left the salon feeling depressed.

Next, we were on to the salons at the mall. We walked into the expensive, supposedly upscale salon front entry and they pretty much kicked us out.

"We do not do tours, nor do we have students come through!" said the snotty Sassoon cut, black-haired woman, pursing her red lipsticked lips.

We never did make it into the trendy salon to tour, and I didn't really care. I knew their *style* was not for me. No pun intended!

A little deflated by now, we headed down the escalator and straight to Montgomery "Monkey" Wards. The salon was placed in the middle of the store, so that meant no windows in the salon. In fact, there was not even a door into the salon, just an opening to walk through.

Blonde Spit Fire was so excited. She was acting as if she owned the joint. The manager who was originally from Peru was welcoming and she looked well put together, not too tall, but a handsome woman. There was another young woman at a station cutting a young man's hair. She turned with a smile and said "Hi everyone." She had a head full of brown curls.

The manager then led us past five stations that were pretty tight, in fact, there was not enough room for us all to fit. We saw the back room with three shampoo bowls and a small two-butt dispensary (where only two stylist butts could fit).

The Peruvian manager spoke in a strong accent, and she told us that this salon was owned by a corporation, and that they paid their employees on a commission basis. Stylists either got minimum wage, which at the time was $3.05 an hour, or 50 percent commission. That was a pretty common way to pay back then.

At the upscale, mod and swanky salon it was different; stylists had to pay to rent their stations. Monthly, they would pay for their space, and also pay for any products or supplies needed: perm solutions, shampoo or the back bar of the color/tint/dye etc.

Ms. Peruvian was pleasant and knew her stuff. Spit Fire was so excited she could hardly contain herself. The Peruvian showed Spit Fire the station where she would be working. The salon was decorated in the 70s trend of oranges and browns. It needed to be updated badly.

I didn't share Spit Fire's enthusiasm, but I tried to not let it show. My thought as we left—*this is the last place I want to work.*

LESSON LEARNED
Just because you get educated does not mean you make tons of money.

MY FINAL HEROIC HAIRCUT

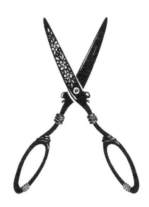

"Number 56" is called for the last time. It felt unreal as I went to the front to grab my very last client in Beauty College. Her name was Henrietta, and she was a beautiful Hispanic woman with gorgeous skin. She was maybe fifty, but in wonderful shape. She looked classy; she dressed wonderfully and made everyone around her take a second look.

As we arrived at the chair, I told her she was my very last client to sit in this chair. *I was graduating!*

She asked me what I was going to do afterwards. With that question, for the first time it dawned on me that I hadn't thought ahead. I'm more of a wake up in the morning—and wait to see what happens kind of person.

"I don't really know." I told her, "I will work in a salon… somewhere!" At eighteen, I didn't think past the current day, even when it came to where I might get a job.

As usual, I started with the consultation. "Are you looking for a new look?" I asked Hot Henrietta. She kind of hemmed and hawed. She said she really wanted to do an above the shoulder length bob.

"Perfect," I agreed. "It will be flirty, and swing when you move. That will be a good look for you."

Hot Henrietta was presently wearing a shoulder length grown out shag, which had no shape. I asked if she had ever heard of an A-Line Bob. I explained, "This is when the hair is cut right at the hairline in the back and longer in the front, resting at about your shoulders. It moves when you move and looks very stylish."

"Perfect," she responded with excitement.

I went to work. I took my time and it was, in fact, a perfect cut. Next, I brought out the mousse, which at the time was a new styling product. Before mousse, there was only Dippy Do gel. Today, hairdressers choose from thousands of new and inventive styling products.

I applied the mousse and used a round brush to blow dry her hair after giving her the best cut that I had ever mastered. She looked impressed and I genuinely felt terrific about accomplishing this cut for her, too.

Hot Henrietta was beaming. She loved it. I told her that I needed to get an instructor's approval, and then we'd be done.

She said, "Okay," as she moved closer to the mirror to run her hands through her great new haircut. I glanced back at my masterpiece, because it is looking fabulous, even from afar.

I had trouble finding an available instructor until

Six-Foot-Two walked over and asked, "Do you want me to help you with the last check?"

I was hesitant to have him take control of anything after the bleach snafu disaster. I tried to avoid him. Besides, he was high most the time.

"Okay," I said. I knew it was a good cut, and afterall, I was a senior! He will just run his comb through it and that would be it. BUT NO! Instead, he immediately started cutting.

Even Hot Henrietta was like "NO!"

His scissors snipped away, and my perfect haircut was no longer an A-Line Bob. He had cut her front the same length as the back. FUCK! What the hell was this high mother scratcher working in a teaching position for? I had no idea!

Well, to tell you the truth, Six-Foot-Two was fired shortly after that. I heard from some of the other students that he was caught with a young female student doing lines of meth in his car. I knew he was bad news in more ways than one.

LESSON LEARNED
Trust your instincts about people, whatever position they hold. Your instincts are usually right!

Kimberly McBee

GRADUATION FINALE

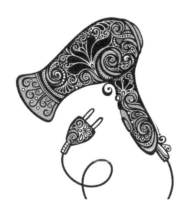

I graduated on a Friday. Done. Completed. Finished!

I soon realized this was advancement, but without any recognition or special commencement!

Mrs. John the head cheese of the the college, unceremoniously gave me my diploma, and I punched out on the time clock and that was that. No walking with my class. No ceremony. Nothing. Not sure what I expected, but I thought it would be more than it was.

Lucky me! One of the new instructors, an older woman with power trip issues, stayed on my case that whole day. She was like a terrier nipping at my heels wherever I was and whatever I was doing.

I didn't sit. I didn't take breaks. She wanted to get as much out of me as possible. It's all about money, and they make money off the students.

Even so, I do think Faye was sad to see me go, because we had bonded. The funny (and kind of sad) thing was I never saw her again. Not once, I saw the other instructors around town after starting in the real work world, but never Faye.

All the students graduate at different times, depending on the time they have spent, hours they have clocked, and the testing they take and pass. Spit Fire graduated the day before me and was the first graduate in our "Lucky 13" class. I was the second to graduate, and after that I don't know. I never set foot back in the school until I was looking for employees for my own salon.

The time finally came for me to punch out on the time clock for the very last time—after fourteen months and one day, because I was sick one day.

I left and never looked back.

LESSON LEARNED
Time to become a grown up!

DON'T DELAY—GET ON WITH LIFE

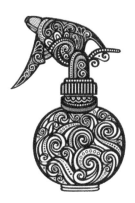

On Monday morning, I awoke to my mother standing over me "Kim, it's time to get up and get ready to go get your license."

To be sure everything stayed fresh in my mind, I had made a reservation to take my test with the state as soon as I graduated. Today was the day! We drove one hour to the state capital in Salem, Oregon.

Without any unexpected "happenings," I took my test and passed—thank God. I would have been so embarrassed to have failed.

My mother was proud, which felt really good to me. And when she was happy, that meant that she would reward me with food, a good meal which always included ice cream. We ate and chatted, and then headed home.

The next day, I got a call from Spit Fire and she was so excited about me passing my test that she could hardly speak.

She quickly asked, "Do you want to work together? The shop I'm going to be working in has an open station."

I tend to have a calm nature, so I thought about it for a minute, then smiled and said, "Sure, why not."

I cringed some, because this shop was the *last* salon I really wanted to work in, because it was old-fashioned and lacked pizzazz, but still, I told myself I could give it my best shot.

At the same time, I appreciated that this was going to be the first salon I got the pleasure to start in. I didn't take this first "station" for granted, and I appreciate that first job to this day.

LESSON LEARNED
Expect the unexpected.

MY FIRST DAY ON THE JOB

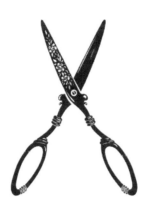

I walked into the Montgomery Wards Salon for my interview. I was greeted by the Peruvian woman who had given us the tour the day we had visited as students.

She smiled, and I noticed that she looked impeccable. I smiled back and shook her hand. She showed me to her office where I asked her a few questions and in return she did the same. It was more like a comfortable conversation.

For my first interview, it was pretty laid back. My breathing became more relaxed, but not for long—because without hesitating, she said I could start on Monday. That was when I began to feel the panic start to rise up within me.

This was a grownup commitment and the end of my freedom. No more summers off. No more late nights and sleeping in. No more childhood. In that moment, I knew I was heading into the unknown world of adult responsibilities, and hoped I was ready.

Monday came too fast. I woke up and hit the shower. I noticed that it was early, but I realized it wasn't any earlier than when I had to get ready for school.

The worry I was feeling could be seen on my face. This was a job that impacted people and how they felt about themselves, and how others saw them. I hoped I could be really good at it, because people would be paying me money to help them look good.

It felt surreal to know that soon my first client would walk in the salon, and sit in my chair, and be paying for my services in a real working environment. I was responsible! It was up to me. No instructor was going to be checking my work.

Of course, this made me think of instructor Six-Foot-Two, so this would be a good thing!

That first morning, my drive to work was about thirty-one minutes, but who was counting? *Me!*

I parked my mother's big red LTD station wagon in a back parking spot by the river, where I was told employees were allowed to park. From way back there, I carried all my beauty school issued equipment into the mall, finally getting to "Monkey" Wards.

A mall security guard held the door for me; my arms felt like they were going to fall off. I arrived on time for my very first day, and I noticed there was already a man sitting in the small, rather stark, but tidy waiting area.

A woman with brown permed curls was at the

front desk. She smiled and said a friendly, "Good Morning."

I smiled back as I greeted her.

She asked, "Would you like to do a walk-in haircut? I would do it, but I have a 9:00 a.m. appointment this morning."

I gave her a look, like—*your kidding right?*

I could see that she was dead serious, so I asked for a few minutes to set up. My calm was only in my words of agreement, because inside I was in a bit of panic and my exterior had started to sweat.

Without hesitating longer, I dashed to my station before I dropped all my curlers, shears and clippers that were piled in my arms.

I threw everything in my station cupboard, without thought of what or where. Feeling this disorganized was not how I envisioned starting my first day on my first job.

The radio was playing quietly... and I'll never forget the song... "Money for Nothing," by Dire Straits.

Finding a drape, I walked with it in my hand to greet the little middle-aged man. He still wore his hat as he sat in the tiny waiting room.

I held out my hand and said, "Hello, my name is Kim. I will be cutting your hair today."

Obviously, he saw me walk in with my hands full of equipment. I'm sure he knew that this was my first day on the job. Before taking him back, I had made a point of setting my state license in the forefront on my station, so he would see that I'm legal. I felt proud to display my accomplishment.

His name was Donald, and I will never forget

him, because he was the first paying client to sit down in my chair—and I stood tall *behind the chair* as I began the consult (just like I would continue to do for decades to come with my clients.)

I started to drape him. First, I put a paper strip around his neck—state regulation. I then said to Donald, "Well, I think you know that this is my first day on the job?" He replied that he had guessed that.

To boost his confidence in me, I told him, "I have been doing this for a while." I sort of lied… *a little.*

He asked if this was my first job out of school, since he had seen me carry my big black suitcase in, along with the other school supplies I juggled. And of course, the suitcase had *Springfield College of Beauty* etched on it. I sort of blushed and admitted that I was caught—this was my first day, and my first job out of school.

Donald took off his hat and said to me, "No worries you can't screw this up!"

This was my lucky day, because under that derby hat he was wearing no hair; he had no hair at all on top! Poor Donald had male pattern baldness.
I sighed with relief. This was going to be an easy cut, and besides, Donald was such a nice guy to help me feel at ease.

After giving Donald a superbly nice haircut, I took him back to the shampoo bowl and gave him a great head massage and conditioned his scalp. He was happy—and so was I!

I went back to my station to retrieve his hat and met him at the front desk. He paid six dollars for his thirty minute haircut and shampoo, and tipped me two dollars. I thought to myself, I have chosen the right profession. I made him happy, I did a good job and I got a tip to prove it.

LESSON LEARNED
The job that makes you happy is the right job.

Kimberly McBee

PLAYING THE FIELD

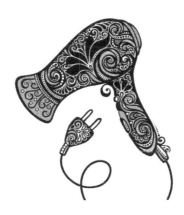

I was a fan of boys! *If only I had known then what I know now.* I dated several boys, not men. I went out with someone different once a week. My mother called it, "playing the field."

I had one boyfriend in high school for three years, and then dated Logan steadily for six months in Beauty College. But I had always liked a nice guy that I had held hands with in sixth grade.

His name was Mike, and he was blonde and had interesting greenish eyes. Not my normal type. I'm more attracted to the dark-haired, dark-skinned, tall, yummy type. Got the picture?

But Mike and I would run into each other, and we could always talk and easily understand each other, (more at ease if you will).

We officially dated for a time after I graduated, but he was still attending a university four hours south of where I was living, but we continued to keep in contact. When he did come home to visit, we would hook up. We were both dating others and there were no strings attached. We were good friends.

One time when he came home, he told me about dating another hairdresser. She was having some trouble. He told me, how recently, she had been cutting a man's hair, and she looked down at the cape that covered his lap, and it was moving up and down, up and down.

She was shocked, because she assumed he was playing with himself while she was doing her job. She took out her hair dryer and without a word, proceeded to hit him with a strong blow to the head. He yelled, "WHAT WAS THAT FOR?"

Upset, she said, "Because you sick bastard, you are jerking off in my chair!" He lifted the cape to show her he was not *playing* with himself, but cleaning his eye glasses!

Shortly after that happened, he pressed charges for assault. I'm not sure how her career as a hairdresser turned out…

LESSON LEARNED
Better know before you blow.

Lessons Learned Behind the Chair

THE "BOB" FROM HELL

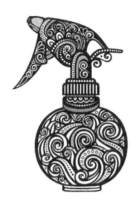

I was working late. We closed at 8 p.m. and it was two hours until closing. A mature lady walked in with her daughter who was in her forties.

I was at the front desk going over my day, which had been very productive. I looked up and greeted them, "Hello, How can I help you?"

The older one of the two said that her daughter would like a haircut. I looked at her daughter and asked her name. She looked at her mother and then back at me before she told me her name was Sam.

Sam's hair did not look like it was in bad shape. In fact, it looked pretty good. I walked her back to my station and prepped her for her service. Her mother sat right behind us in one of the dryer chairs. If I were to take two steps back I would have stepped on her toes. I started my consult. I asked what she would like to do and if she wanted to go shorter?

Again, Sam first looked at her mother and then back

at me. They looked like professionals; I surmised that they worked in an office or maybe one of the jewelry stores in the mall. Not low end, more high end clothing, make up, nice jewelry and expensive shoes.

To my question, Sam hesitated, and responded with, "Mom how short should I cut it?" Her mother decided she should just take off one-half of an inch, keeping it in the same style.

Easy enough. I cut it and in twenty minutes I was finished. It looked good, not much different, but good.

Sam looked at it in the mirror and said, "Well, I think I want another one-half inch off. I was finished, and had to start all over. "No problem" I said calmly. Back then, I had lots and lots of patience. Without comment, I did as she asked.

I finished for the second time and her mother piped in, "Maybe another one-half inch?"

I looked at her and said in my head… *really?*

This time, I specifically asked Sam if she wanted to go even shorter and she agreed. I noticed that the expression on her face didn't look like it was what she really wanted, so I asked to make sure this was what she wanted. I knew this was going to be my last and final time cutting this same head of hair.

To help her visualize it, I asked "Would you like the ends to be right under your chin?" She said "I think so."

Time was ticking away, getting closer to our 8:00 p.m closing time. Breathing to calm myself, I started again. I was the only one still working, Peruvian was in the back room cleaning and eating a snack.

I cut Sam's hair for the third time, and it was a perfect chin length bob. She looked at it when I finished and asked, "What do you think if I go shorter? I thought she was talking to me, but quickly I realized she was asking mommy. Mommy looked at her and said, "Yes, by all means go shorter."

I asked, trying not to show my frustration, "How much shorter this time?"

"Take it just below my ears, so I can still tuck it behind them."

I explained that the back would have to be shorter than the front, or at this length it would look like a bowl cut or a Dutch boy. She said, even without looking at mommy, "I'm okay with that."

Number four here we go! I cut a pretty little a-line bob to just below her ears. And it was 7:55 p.m. and the salon was supposed to close in five minutes.

I finished with, what by now, had to be a masterpiece. She looked in the mirror and back again at her mother. I stopped them in their tracks, saying, "The shop closes in five minutes and four haircuts is the max I am willing to do at this time."

They both said nothing as they began to evaluate the cut in the mirror—and before one more word was spoken from either of them, I ripped off the cape draping from Sam's body and started for the front desk.

I waited for them as they got up. Their body language spoke loud and clear, as if I was the one in the wrong. They got all snooty.

I told them that it would be six dollars. Now that I

think of it, I regret that I didn't have the nerve to charge them for each cut. They proceeded to slap down six one dollar bills and left in a huff. By then, I was tired (of them) and really wanted to scream.

Instead, I sat down, filled out my time sheet and cleaned my station. It would be ready for my day again at 9:00 a.m.

LESSON LEARNED
At some point you need to cut the cord!

MOVING OUT!

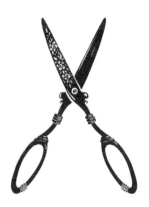

My mother was amazing, after raising two kids before me, and one that was eight years younger, she had gotten pretty relaxed. I lived at home, but could come and go as I pleased. I was nineteen and had no cares in the world. I had just started my new career, so had a little money, too.

Wide-Eyed Curly Hair, from beauty school, was raised by much stricter parents. She called me one day, "Can you meet for lunch?"

"Sure," I said, "I would be happy to." It was Monday and my day off. I hopped into my car, which was at the time a 1980 Mustang.

Sidenote: My grandparents had taken pity on me after I wrecked my first car. They knew I was using my mother's car, which was inconvenient. They went with me to test drive a few cars.

The Mustang was not my choice, but I showed up at my grandparent's home one day and they had it sitting in their garage. It was kind of hard to tell them I didn't really want it.

My wrecked Plymouth had been parked at their home for a year. One day they called and said they were tired of it sitting on their property, and that I needed to get it ready to sell. They sounded mean.

I was upset when I arrived at their place. During their call, they did not act like the loving grandparents that they normally were. They told me to come out there and vacuum and clean the Plymouth.

When I got to their house, they said that I could find the vacuum in their big shop, so I stomped out to the big shop. When I walked in, I saw the Mustang that we had test driven. I almost dropped to my knees. I started to cry, and I ran back up the stairs at their house to hug them both.

Not so fast! That is when the stipulations began. My grandmother told me that I would need to pay them back three thousand dollars. They had a contract set up. I was to pay them one hundred and fifty dollars each month until the three thousand owing them was paid off.

If the old Plymouth sold, I could put that money towards the Mustang. My Grandma also said I had to be home by ten o'clock in the evening. She knew this was her chance to use the car as leverage to keep me following some of my mom's rules and help keep me out of trouble.

I agreed to the contract, because I had a job that could cover this payment. It would take only two weeks' worth of pay each month.

Back to meeting Wide-Eyed Curly Hair—I drove my gold-colored hatch-back Mustang to meet her. We met at the mall at Darby Donuts. Wide-Eyed

Curly Hair explained that her mother was being too strict. She was nineteen and had a curfew of ten o'clock.

She had worked hard in a bakery, before and while in Beauty College. She had saved everything she made and wanted to move out. She was working for Perfect Look Salon, and still worked in the bakery on the days she was not in the salon. She needed a roommate.

I thought about it and said, "Why not?"

We both decided to look at places in nearby towns and see what we could come up with. I took Springfield, where we went to college. She took Eugene, where we both worked. The two towns run into each other, separated by a river and Interstate 5. They are just a few miles apart.

Wide Eyed showed me three options. The first one had a manager of the apartment building that was scary looking: nasty teeth and the male version of the manager of *Kingpin* (the movie). I felt that he looked at us two young girls like fresh meat, especially since there were street walkers, drug dealers and panhandlers in the area. I thought about this place for about two seconds and told her this one was off the list for sure.

The next one that she had found in Eugene was a two-story house and we could rent the top story. The top-story apartment had a claw foot tub next to the side wall in the front room. *Seriously?*

If that was not bad enough, there was a homeless shack in the back yard. I told her I would not feel comfortable bathing without walls—and in the front room at that! I also did not feel good about the area, plus the two dudes that lived downstairs were staring at us through their window. They looked like serial killers. After this, I decided not to even see her third option. She was going to be surprised with what I had come up with in Springfield for the same price.

I took her to an apartment building that was in a safe area where lots of university students lived. There was an in-ground pool and even a playground for children. The available two bedroom apartment had one bath on the bottom floor. I also liked it because it had a covered patio with a view of the pool. She was loving it, too.

There were young people living there, and nicer cars in the parking area—much more my speed. We talked to the manager. She was an older lady that was fairly nice. She introduced herself as Marge, and was excited that we were interested. Wide Eyes handed her the first and last month's rent and the cleaning fee before we left.

Without even giving it any thought, I moved out of my parent's house. I just did it.

LESSON LEARNED
Being spontaneous can lead you down a different path.

FRIENDSHIP LOST

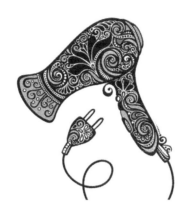

Spitfire and I had gone to Beauty College together and now we were working together, with our stations right next to each other. I watched all her clients come and go. I did haircuts, and began to collect repeat clientele. I did not see this same thing happening for Spitfire. I actually heard patrons come in and ask *not* to get her again.

The woman that was working with me, Curls, was well liked and was a good stylist. She seemed to collect men, mostly. She was a flirt. She rubbed her breasts on her male clients while she was blow drying. She was tipped well. Hmm…

Few days were dull from my observation point. A woman came in to get a perm one day from Spit Fire. She not only soaked her from the collar to her underwear, but the curl did not take. She then had to start returning money for her work. Obviously Ms. Peruvian never liked to return money. This did not make her look good.

Not looking good, Spitfire came in late one morning after I had already opened. I had already apologized to her first client that was waiting in the tiny waiting area. In fact, she raced to the back and threw up in the sink. I went back and asked her if I could help. She shooed me away with her hand.

I decided to take on her client to help her. My client was not due for about fifteen minutes. I introduced myself and escorted Phillis to my chair. She had never been in before, so I consulted with her and did the trim she requested. Phillis was accommodating, and left after paying for her cut.

She didn't mention the sickly girl in the back, and she even tipped me my first $5.00 tip ever. I thanked her and sent her happily on her way...

Spitfire was still in the back and not feeling well. Her skin was white as a ghost, and I really started worrying about her.

Peruvian came in later, since she was working the closing shift that evening. She saw Spitfire looking sick and uncomfortable. She took her into the back room, and when Spitfire came out she looked pissed off.

Without a word to anyone, I saw Spitfire collect her items. She was taking everything she owned, leaving nothing of hers at the shop. Until that day, I had no idea she was pregnant. Clearly, morning sickness is not for wimps.

Years later I ran into Spitfire. I had assumed that she had quit that day because she was pregnant. But Ms. Peru had actually fired her. I never knew that's what had happened. I learned from Spitfire that she had never forgiven me since that day she had to leave. It was a complete misunderstanding. I shared with her that I hadn't known that she had been fired.

I've not seen her since that day we ran into each other. It's sad that a friendship can be broken due to lack of communication.

LESSON LEARNED
Ask questions, don't always assume!

Kimberly McBee

1980s—PERM RAGE!

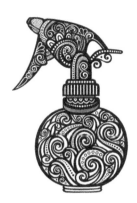

Perm's! Perm's! Perm's! We permed everyone.

The youngest client I permed was three years old, and oldest was one hundred and three. She was quite a lady—with fourteen grandchildren.

One day, a new client, Connie walked in with her daughter, who was in elementary school. I would guess she was around eight or nine years old, and Connie, her mother, wanted to have a perm put in her hair.

She was the oldest child in her family. I took her back to the chair. I asked her name, as she settled in on the booster seat I'd put in my hydraulic chair.

"My name is Jamie! I'm eight and I want curly hair!" Right then, I knew she was one that knew exactly what she wanted. My perfect client!

I wrapped her hair in a spiral design. (This is a vertical wrap of the curlers, candlestick like.)

The wrap took a couple of hours because little

Jamie had tons of hair. She was getting tired and becoming a little brat in the process. Her mom had left for two hours to shop and I began to feel like a babysitter the more she began to act out.

I finally finished the wrap. I put the chemicals that smell to high heaven on each curler. By now, Jamie was getting loud, "This stuff stinks. "I don't want to do this anymore." I kept telling her that we were almost done. It will be worth it.

Maybe she wasn't feeling it, because she started to cry. I calmed her down and gave her a lollipop. About that time Connie, Jamie's mother had got back, carrying five big bags. She had been having fun with her free time to shop the entire mall. .

And what about me? *I was pulling my hair out* as I rinsed the little princess. I then took her back to the salon chair. She started calming down some, while I stood behind the chair, combing her hair out.

At last, I was done, and she looked in the mirror and I could tell she was excited about the look. I have to admit she was a pretty little girl, and the Shirley Temple curls looked adorable.

Connie was pleased. We went to the front desk and checked out. Connie asked me when she could get in for a perm.

I asked her if she had brought Jamie in as a guinea pig. Connie smiled. She said her neighbor had told her about me. Then, after seeing Jamie's hair, she confessed that she had put her daughter in the chair first to decide if she wanted to sit there herself for a perm. Now there's a smart woman!

I started doing Connie's perms and hair in 1986 and I still do her hair today. Oh, and Jamie grew into a nice young woman who now has little ones of her own.

LESSON LEARNED
Some clients become like family.

Kimberly McBee

COWORKER CRAZINESS

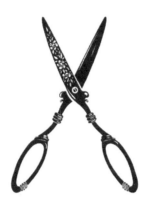

Working alongside other women, and even men, you really have to be tolerant. In close quarters, there is the reality that some coworkers behave differently and are louder than others.

Brown Curls was my first experience with another stylist that loved her work. She was engaged, and was just plain sexy. Her big brown eyes and curly brown hair gave her an exotic look. She stood about five feet eight and wore heels to boot.

One day a young man came in and she ended up with him in her chair. I had a break, so I sat in my own styling chair to watch her work. You can learn a lot from watching others who have been in the trade awhile.

However, what I saw was not what I expected. She was touching him tenderly, treating him like she was attracted to him. She giggled and flirted, making him blush. Brown Curls was well into her early thirties and the client in her chair was about twenty.

I was almost embarrassed watching this going on. I was not a fan of what she was up to, due to the fact that she was engaged to another man. Things thickened between them over time. This 20-year-old guy came around to see Brown Curls at least three to four times a week and not just to get haircuts. They started going to lunch together, and going out together when her fiancé was out of town.

Brown Curls confessed to me she was having sexual relations with the 20-year-old—and that she was his first sexual partner. I couldn't believe she would do this to her fiancé, much less tell me!

She had no thought of breaking things off. She was still planning her wedding while screwing this youngster.

I was not only feeling sorry for her fiancé, but also for the young guy who at some point she would break it off with. He was definitely in lust.

Twenty-year-old even stood outside the huge doors that entered into the main store and watched Brown Curls work. He reminded me of a stalker. I was even a little freaked out and he was not watching me.

She finally got the courage to tell him she needed to break it off, and she made him go a little crazy. That was when the stalking really began.

She confessed it all to her fiancé, and he had "a talk" with 20-year-old. After that, we never saw him hanging around the store again.

All I have to say is that she must have been good in bed because her fiancé never blinked an eye. He just went with it.

But… I wonder… maybe she never really confessed to him as much about it as she told me she did.

LESSON LEARNED
Cougars come in all ages.

Kimberly McBee

STUPID IS AS STUPID DOES

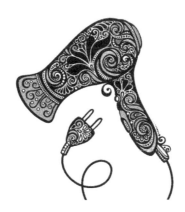

A new coworker, Spanish speaking, tall and talented at short hair, was hired where I worked. She was able to speak two languages, and that made me jealous.

However, as far as a stylist, I noticed people should not sit in her chair unless they wanted short hair! She once cut my hair two inches *short* on top, I felt like Rod Stewart. Not a good look on me with my round face and five-foot-five frame.

One day the phone rang and Spanish Speaking answered. "Hello! Yes, this is a salon. Yes, Kim works here."

The way she said my name—*KEEEM* was kind of cute. On the call, she went on to say, "Sure"… "Keeem, you're wanted on the phone."

I walked to the front desk. I discovered after answering the phone and telling me I was wanted on the phone, Spanish Speaking had then hung it up, ending the call.

I then asked Spanish Speaking, "I thought I was wanted on the phone?"

She looked at me and then the phone and shrugged like nothing was wrong. She did not say "I'm sorry, I'm an idiot" or even apologize. Not a word of explanation, as if she had done nothing wrong. I walked away shaking my head, in disbelief.

And then there was Bonnie. The day she walked in, it was as if she had befriended me in a former life. We clicked!

She took over Spitfire's old station, next to mine. She was an excellent stylist. She knew color and taught me a few new tricks.

Bonnie had cool hair like a rock star—permed, colored and big. My hair at that point was bleached almost white and permed and back combed; big band hair. Bonnie's was longer than mine and reddish brown in the back and blonde in the front. She had her own style, for sure.

Working together, was a match made in heaven. She was fun and loved her job, as I did. One evening while we were finishing up, she closed out the till and put the change bag with the full cash deposit for all the stylists that day on the front counter. The total was just under five hundred dollars.

Bonnie left it and walked into the back room to hit the lights. I was working at my station, setting it up for the next day's work. I came out and she jokingly asked me, "What did you do with the bag?"

I replied, "What? I don't know what you're talking about."

Sounding tense, she said "The bank bag. Stop joking around Kim."

"I really don't know what you are talking about." I answered.

Come to find out, someone walked by just as she put the bag on the counter—in the blink of an eye, someone grabbed the bag, and you guessed it, Bonnie was fired over it. They never caught who did it.

But that was not cool. I was now the assistant manager and helping with payroll, so I was more engrossed in the dollars and cents of the salon. No extra pay for the "title," so I really had no reason to stay on, but I did have a hard time leaving Peru.

Before making my decision to move salons, Spanish Speaking told me she was opening a shop across from the mall. I thought about it, but having observed her lack of business sense, I decided to not take her up on it.

LESSON LEARNED
Don't let your guard down.

Kimberly McBee

JENNY'S CRIME

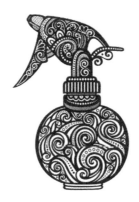

Remember Jenny, my friend from high school that I would go to dance clubs with, while in Beauty College? One workday, she came to meet me for lunch.

The week before, Jenny and I were at a party, and Bonnie, my coworker who had just been fired at the salon (the previous story), told Jenny how she would shoplift at one of the major stores in the mall, and then return the stolen items for cash. Not at all cool!

I listened silently as Bonnie talked. Her *skill* included shoplifting designer jeans because they sold or returned for over 100 dollars a pop.

Before meeting me for lunch, (Jenny told me later) that she had taken an empty cotton purse into the store Bonnie told her about. She went into a dressing room that was not monitored and stuffed two pair of jeans, a sweater, and two sets of leggings into her purse.

I remember her telling me that she even put in a few tank tops. As she attempted to leave the store, she was seen by the undercover security.

At the time, I was working and just about ready to take my lunch break to meet her, since we had plans to go to lunch. Little did I know that on the other side of the mall, she had been taken by security, and was being retained in the store she had been caught stealing from.

I got called to the phone at the front desk of my work. "Hello, this is Kim."

A deep male voice speaks, "Can you tell me who this person is?"

It was Jenny he put on the phone. "Tell them who I am, Kim!"

I recognized her voice, and the deep male voice took the receiver again, and asked me if I could identify her. I told him that her name was Jenny. Then the phone went dead.

I was terrified. I did not know if she had been kidnapped. I did not have any idea what was going on. Ten minutes went by and I finished my clean up not knowing what to do since I had no idea who had called, or what the call was about. Remember, this was before caller ID or cell phones. I had no way to track the call.

About the time I finished cleaning up, Jenny walked into the salon in a panic. "I was so scared."

I asked her who had called and what was going on. She told me what she had done. Then she told me how they had dragged her into a back room and questioned her for an hour. They wanted to know where she learned how to do this. She didn't have any ID on her, so she could not prove who she was, that is why they called me.

The department store ended up suing Jenny and took her to court. She did not drive, so I took her to the courthouse. I sat with her, not because I agreed with what she had done, but just to be a supportive friend.

I'll never forget her standing up when they called her name. They stated why she was there, and named the crime they felt she had committed.

The judge asked if she was pleading guilty or not guilty. Jenny said in a shaky voice, "NOT GUILTY."

The judge, sitting up above us, in his black robe said, "You will need to hire a lawyer and we will set a date for your next court date."

Jenny panicked. "I'll have to hire a lawyer?"

"Yes, that is how this works, Miss."

Jenny changed her verdict. The courthouse, full of people waiting to be called up, went into hysterics. Everyone was cracking up, including me.

She began confessing. We were seated among drug addicts, motorcycle gangs with their tattooed skin and leathers, and a lady who looked like she worked the corners to make her living. I could not wait to get out of there. This was not my idea of an interesting, fun, new experience.

The judge told Jenny that she was being fined $300 dollars and the department store had the right to claim additional compensation as well, up to $800 dollars. She would also have to visit the city jail for a *tour*—the date and time would all be arranged for her!

Without pause, "Do I get to keep the clothes?" Jenny asked seriously. The laughter started again. Not from me—I was sitting in total amazement. I loved Jenny, but she could be dumber than a bag of hammers!

We walked to my car and Jenny said something I will never forget. "They did not even let me have the stuff I stole!"

Some people never learn—and I knew it was pointless to give my opinion, so I didn't.

I saw her years later and she was the same. She had a small son. Jenny was also static working a few part time jobs and still lived in an apartment. She had thumbtacked pictures on her apartment walls, with no frames, just like we did as teens. This really kind of stumped me. Sadly, I guess it was symbolic of her state of maturity.

LESSON LEARNED
Takes all kinds in this world.

FOILING IN THE 80s

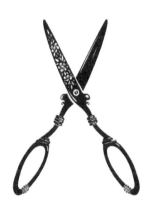

I was working in the mid-eighties in Eugene, Oregon when foiling hair was just starting—this is when aluminum foil took on a newfangled meaning for me, and it became more valuable.

Montgomery Wards had a cafeteria with a buffet. All of the anchor stores, like JC Penny's, Meier and Frank, and Montgomery Ward's had cafeterias back then. I could smell mashed potatoes and gravy while working *or* shopping. It was a short walk to the cafeteria, since it was only about fifty feet from my salon. The smell of the buffet reminded me not only of hunger pangs, but of my need for foil as I began to master the new foiling technique on my clients.

I got to know the lunch lady, and talked sweetly to her. She was not the friendliest. (I always wonder about those types of women. As a young woman, I imagined that they still lived with their elderly mothers and were all old maids. Those that I observed never wore make-up and never dressed in anything but hair nets and colorless clothing, complemented with military-like shoes.)

I talked sickeningly sweet; I admit it, so that I could borrow tin foil from the stash that they kept in the back. The box was about forty pounds, so back then I figured they could spare some.

She would give me a big box of foil, intended for leftovers or to cover dishes, and I would pack it back to the salon to use for hair creations. I would hide out in the back room of the salon and fight with the huge box on top of the clothes dryer, as I cut the foil into neat little rectangular shapes. Hundreds of them!

I "foiled" anyone I could, as it became an innovative new trend. I loved highlighting and refused to torture people with the frosting cap and crochet hook any more.

Sonja is my funniest memory; a great example of the intrigue of foiling in the early years. She came to me one day and said she was Hawaiian and Japanese, and that she had always wanted lighter hair, but knew she would not look good totally blonde.

I told her about how weaving worked. "We could highlight your hair, then put color over the top and give you a lighter look without looking cheap or with one dramatic color change."

She was willing and liked the idea. We started. I got out my thick "cafeteria" foils and started foiling her beautiful virgin black hair. I put bleach within the folded foil, to lighten her hair to a pale yellow. When I was done the thick foils were so massive that she had a head three feet wide and four feet tall. During the process, she made it fun for me because she was so excited she couldn't stop smiling.

Sonya was a manager in one of the grocery stores in Eugene. She was married and had two small children. Sometimes these types of women, who work hard raising kids and are married, never get pampered. She was like so many women who always give themselves to others day-in and day-out. This sucks their time and energy.

I went into the back dispensary to choose the color to put on top. This would tone the precise highlights. I walked back in after choosing a cinnamon toner. I held back my laughter. She looked adorable with the huge head of foils and her perm-a-grin.

She loved my color suggestion, so I took her to the shampoo bowl and we rinsed the bleach down the drain. I'm glad she *could not* see her hair before I toned it. It was bright canary yellow. She looked like a bumble bee. I quickly toned it with the warm cinnamon and she looked fabulous. I practically skipped her back to my chair to style it. I had cut her hair three weeks before, so there was no cut needed. After styling, she was so excited she hugged me, practically laying a sloppy kiss on me.

The hair, each of us wear on our head is such a personal thing. I'm honored that people wear my art every day. Her joy and excitement over her hair made me so happy.

The next time I colored Sonya's hair, she was going to a costume party. I asked, "What are you going as?"

Low and behold, she told me she was going to be a bumble bee! I told her I had a wonderful, fun idea. "You should let me do the first foil and bleach process and wear it like that with your costume. Then Tuesday, come back in and get the toning done! You will literally have black and yellow hair if we do that."

I added, "If you don't like the look, we can go ahead and tone it today."

We foiled and rinsed and then walked back to the chair to cut her hair. She was laughing at her reflection. She decided to wait to tone it.

I told her that I would come in on Monday to tone it, even though it was my day off. She proudly walked out with her black and yellow bumble bee hair.

I secretly hoped nobody asked her who did it.

LESSON LEARNED
What we won't do to win a prize!

GETTING CAUGHT IN THE MIDDLE

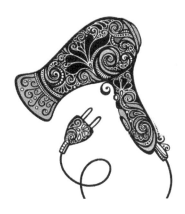

A Native American, young, with long black hair walked in the salon. I was sitting at the desk hoping another victim would walk in since I was having a slow day.

He asked about getting a perm. I told him I could do it immediately. He said he worked at the toy store in the mall. "Let me tell my manager, real quick." He ran out and was back in no time. I draped him and understood he only wanted a perm in the back and wanted to keep all the length too.

"No problem." I said. We walked to the back, and I shampooed him, and then I got him settled back into the chair at my station. I started to wrap his hair—in not too small, but not too big of rollers.

I was almost ready to apply the perming solution when his wife walked in. She was pregnant. It appeared that his wife, Annie, was ready to have the baby that day. She was carrying that baby straight out in front. I asked if they had other children.

She told me that they had a boy who was one. "Wow, they will be close in age," I remarked, smiling.

As I touched her husband's hair to complete the perm, Annie seemed angry, tired, and jealous. . I continued to work, trying to befriend her, but she would not take down her wall.

I finished the perm. He wanted to leave with his hair wet, so he paid… while dripping.

A few days later, Native American walks in and introduced me to the manager of the toy store. Her name was Annie also. He wanted me to cut her hair. The funny thing was he did not introduce her as Annie; he said "This is my girlfriend, Annie."

He said this in a bragging kind of way. I tried not to give him the satisfaction, by acting shocked, or giving any reaction. I treated her like any other client and said I was pleased to meet her. I led her back to the station. She was pretty and sweet, unlike the other Annie I had met. But I couldn't help feeling sorry for his pregnant wife, Annie.

Girlfriend Annie told me she just wanted a trim, She had fine, beautiful, long hair with a slight wave in it. She looked like she may have been a cheerleader type in high school. I decided to try to make some sense of this odd scenario.

I asked Annie if she had any children. She replied that she had one child and her name was Kimberly. I asked how old and she said that her daughter was one. I continued with my twenty questions. I then asked if she was married, and she told me she was separated. She seemed somewhat satisfied telling me so. By now, I was done cutting her hair and started to blow it dry, and in walked her boyfriend Native American.

"How's it going?" he asked. "Great. She is a new woman," I responded. He paid for her service and they walked off, hand in hand.

A few days later, in walked, Annie, the pregnant wife. Without a *hi* or a *how are you doing,* she said, "I would like to ask you a question."

I said. "Sure, what can I help you with?" I was hoping it was a hair question, but, no, she was in a very vulnerable state, and due any day. She asked me if I had cut a girl's hair yesterday and if her husband had come in with her.

I weighed in on how to answer and just wanted to grab my purse and run, not walk, out the door—and go have a strong cocktail—I didn't like being stuck in the middle. It surprised me what came out of my mouth. I asked. "Annie, do you trust your husband?"

She looked at me and then teary eyed saying "No Kim, I do not trust him."

"I think you know the answer then." I replied. I did not want to tell her, but I also did not want her to be made out to be a fool.

From then on, she became a client and I got to give her little baby girl, who was delivered a few days later, her first haircut. Her two kids are now married and have children of their own.

I saw the cheating bastard years later. He was on the streets begging for a cigarette or a dollar. Neither Annie nor her children have anything to do with him.

If I hadn't known better, I would believe Cheater was on drugs, because of his thin, sunken-in face and red sores on his skin.

LESSON LEARNED
Grass is not always greener on the other side

BRAZEN BEHAVIOR & BLEACHERS

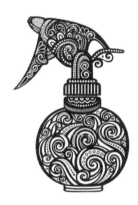

My first apartment, with Wide-Eyed Curly Hair was great. The only problem was keeping up with paying rent. I owed $150 to my grandparents each month and I was bringing in $300 a month.

My rent was $150 a month, and if you do the math I didn't have much left to pay for electricity or food. Wide Eyes had a savings account and she was the generous one who got us into the apartment. I hoped for tips so I could survive on the plus side.

One evening, we had a bunch of friends over and phoned for pizza delivery. The address we gave the pizza man was a couple doors down from us. While the pizza man tried to make his delivery, the guys that were visiting us decided to steal three full pies out of his delivery truck.

We ate very well that night. At the time, I never felt bad. Now I think about that poor guy who was blamed for the loss. Plus, the people who ordered the pizza's got them really late, if they got them at all.

Another time, we went to a fast food restaurant and got a couple burgers and the order was wrong. With the same friends, we decided to lie and tell them the order was way off. We ended up eating ourselves full again. Why was this kind of behavior so fun?

I played volleyball all the time. I would pick up games at the free open gyms around town. I came home late one evening after work and wanted to hit the courts. I went in and Wide Eyes was sitting in the front room of our apartment.

She was there with the neighbors that lived upstairs, whom I chose not to befriend, because they dealt crystal meth. They were cutting bluish white powder on my ugly glass coffee table.

I asked Wide Eyes "What the hell are you doing?" She was so happy.

"You have to try this." She stood up and pushed some of the stuff under my nose.

"No, no I don't!" I screeched

I ran out of the apartment in my shorts and tee shirt and got in my car, hoping these scrungy people would be gone when I got back.

I drove to the gym. I locked my car door and walked in. The gym was busy and there were three courts, all playing games.

I felt good about myself that night. I looked good! My hair was long and still blonde, and I was tan from the Indian summer sun. It was October.

I was sitting all alone up on the top of the

bleachers, even though they were not pulled out. Before I knew it, a guy around my age sat down next to me.

"Hi," he said, in a relaxed friendly manner.
I turned and looked at him and said "Hi" back.

"My name is Mark," he smiled.

"Hi Steve," I said like a smart ass. I wanted to get him to leave me alone. I was there to play volleyball. It was my single focus, and I really didn't want to be picked up.

I was so upset with my stupid roommate who was getting into something she knew nothing about. *(Who thought it up anyway... lets snuff chemicals up our nose?)*

Though my mood was less than inviting, Mark was persistent. He asked if I wanted to play volleyball with him and his friends. He asked politely. I looked and saw there was a girl in the group he was pointing to. I agreed to play.

He introduced his friends to me; Steve and Connie. I thought he was kidding with the "Steve" thing, but no, he was very straight forward. We played a couple games and they were pretty fun to play with.

Not to mention, Mark was a pretty good volleyball player. After we finished playing, Mark asked if I would like to go get a beer with them. By now, I was twenty years old and the last time I checked twenty-one was the legal drinking age.

Mark went on to tell me that we would go over to Connie's house and have a beer. "I'll think about it," I coyly responded.

Interesting, since my mood wasn't the best—but Mark was being very persistent—he even drove up to me as I walked out to my car in the parking lot.

He was driving a little silver sports car with the stereo playing. "Hey, how about that beer?" *I gave in.*

He asked me to follow him, saying that it was not far from where I lived. I never caught on to him knowing where I lived since I had just met him.

I followed the silver sports car and he was right, it was close to my apartment. I got out of my car and walked in, casually, with my sweatshirt tied around my waist.

Connie and Steve were already in the house. Connie's roommate had the crochet hook, and was pulling some poor soul's hair through a frosting cap at the kitchen table. Connie and I talked and I found out that both she and her roommate were stylists. I immediately felt more comfortable.

Connie was twenty-two and Steve was around thirty, with a well manicured beard. Mark was twenty-one. He offered me a beer. I thought, *hey buddy, you are contributing to a minor.* I really didn't like beer, but I sipped on it to be polite, as I watched Connie's roommate turn the girl in the dining room chair a platinum blonde with heavy highlights. She looked like Debbie Harry when she was done—you know, Blondie the new wave, punk rock, singer from the late 70s early 80s.

I kept wondering how they were going to rinse it out. We all talked a little, and when ten o'clock rolled around I told them thanks for the beer. I only had consumed a fourth of it, but headed to my car. Mark ran after me and asked for my number and wanted to know if he could take me out sometime.

"Sure, I answered, never expecting anything to come out of this brief rendezvous.

Surprise! The next day Mark called. He asked if I would like to go out for dinner on Friday night. It was Friday. I asked, "Which Friday? He said, "Tonight!"

He wanted to know if seven o'clock would be okay to pick me up—and I told him it sounded good.

He was so confident. Mark showed up and I realized I never told him where I lived. (I found out later, he had talked to a guy I had dated from the volleyball courts. He asked if it would bother him if he asked me out. No problem, so he gave Mark my phone number and told him where I lived.)

For our date, I dressed in a pink miniskirt and a black top and my famous short, white Bon Jovi boots with tassels. (Remember, it was the 80s—don't judge me.)

I sat next to him in the silver sports car and we drove away with the stereo playing, "Like a Virgin by Madonna." *Perfect song for the occasion.* We arrived at a Chinese restaurant by the water.

We walked in, side-by-side. The woman at the front desk asked if we had reservations. "Yes," Mark said, "for two."

The woman said back, "For *tree*?"

No, Mark says, trying not to laugh, "For two."

We followed the lady back, as she carried the two menus that were bigger than she was. She seated us in a booth.

As soon as we started to talk, she slapped down two glasses of water. I was nervous, and really had no appetite. Mark ordered for both of us. I asked for a coke. She looked at him with this quizzical expression. I did not know he had ordered two cocktails.

I told her to forget the coke. In my limited experience, I had to find someone that was twenty-one to buy my alcohol—and it was something like peach schnapps from the grocery store, that had a three percent alcohol content or something.

Now I was in a regular restaurant with an *older man* with good manners—and he even paid the bill! Thank God, because I would have had to dine and dash.

Little did I know that he would end up being my wonderful husband—this Steve guy!

LESSON LEARNED
You just never know when you'll meet Mr. Right.

DOUBLE BOOKING

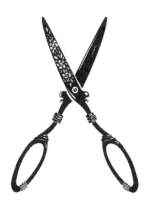

It was Friday and I couldn't wait for the weekend. I worked Saturdays, and to me, there was something fun about working on the weekend. Saturdays always seemed to be so busy and time flew by.

But right now was Friday, and even though it was busy, time was not moving very fast. I was working behind the chair and giving a permanent wave to a lady that worked in a high-end dress shop in the mall.

She was tall and pretty; the type of pretty that would still be gorgeous, even if I shaved her head.

About that time, a man walked in and all the stylists were helping other clients. He kept ringing the bell at the front desk. So I excused myself and went to the front. We had no receptionist.

"Ding!" The bell rang again, even though I knew he could see me coming. This should have been my first clue to the type of person he was.

I asked, "How can I help you?"

The not-so-pretty man asked for, or should I say pleaded for a haircut. I looked around and saw that I was the only one that had a few minutes. I told him that if he could be patient I could work him in, in about three minutes. He looked relieved and sat in the tiny waiting area. Before I headed back to my pretty client, I could already hear his impatient foot tapping.

I went back to the pretty client and finished with a stylist plastic cap, and got her seated under a hooded dryer. I then walked back up to the waiting area and put his name on the books. Brad.

"Brad, follow me please." Brad was walking behind me when I heard him ask, "What is that smell? It stinks in here!"

I told him I had just applied perm solution to another client, to give her curly hair. "Gross, it stinks!"

I thought... *Ya, well, I don't even smell it any longer.* "We do them all day long," I said with a smile. Remember, I was on a time limit, I was doing him a favor by getting him in. (Working in clients is not always the best on my nerves.)

I draped complaining, Badass Brad. I asked him what he would like done. He wanted a trim, so I started to dry cut his hair.

"Aren't you not going to wash my hair?"

I told him the person under the dryer only gave us twenty minutes for his cut. "You are going to rush?" he said in a smart-ass tone.

"No, I'm not going to rush, but you came in without an appointment when we were already busy. So I'm working you in, and I will take the time that we need, but without compromising the client's time that is under the dryer. She made an appointment for her service.

He clearly did not care about the pretty client with the appointment. I walked him back to the shampoo chair.

He sat in the chair and I leaned him back and got a clear look at his face. He was enjoying being an ass. So I put the timer for the pretty client in my pocket and hoped it went off in his ear. I shampooed him and he requested I shampoo him twice. I did as he asked. Now we are really limited on time.

I sat Badass Brad up and used a towel to dry his dripping locks. I walked him back and while I was walking him back to the chair, the timer went off. He just about jumped in the clients lap next to me. I sat him down and told him it was time for me to rinse my perm.

I left Badass Brad and lifted the dryer and saw my pretty clients curls were ready to be rinsed. I walked her back and saw in the mirror that Badass Brad was not happy to have to wait. My pretty client had no clue. I rinsed her, taking my time. She was obviously much more pleasant to be around. I heard, but tried to ignore, Badass Brad's foot again tapping on the floor. After applying warm neutralizer and setting the timer for five minutes I went back to cut Badass Brad. I arrived at my station, and he was clearly annoyed. I cut his hair without saying much, and then dried it in seconds, with two minutes to spare before the time went off. I took the cape off, and he looked amazed. I walked him to the front desk.

He paid, and as he walked out I said, "Have a nice

day!" (I did not add, don't come back! I sure wanted to.)

My pretty client was waiting in the shampoo area and I took off the cotton, which had done its job, keeping the neutralizer from dripping on her face. I rinsed her for the last time and then walked her back to the station with excitement; the curls had come out perfectly.

Pretty loved it. I styled her and walked her out. She paid and tipped me. I told her I would make a record card for her, and gave her my business card. She was a sweetheart.

But before I went back to clean up, Badass Brad came storming in. My look of confusion showed on my face. "I want to see a manager!"

I immediately walked to the back room where Peru was folding some towels, and said, "The man I cut during my perm is back and wants to see a manager."

I started to explain to Peru that he had known that I was squeezing him in.

She said "I watched the whole thing. Just send him back."

I walked up to the front and saw him tapping his boney fingers on the desk. I told him that *the manager* was in the back room and that he could go on back. Badass Brad puffed out his chest and headed to the back.

I heard Peru say "HELLO!"—and then the door shut. I can still hear, "You are a THIEF." Again, louder in almost a shout, "You are a THIEF."

Badass Brad came out of the back with his tail between his legs. I learned later that Peru had given

Brad the tongue lashing of his life. He came in to get his money back and report that I was not a good stylist. He told her I had rushed, and that I did not deserve to work here.

She stuck up for me. She did not cower. I had more respect for her that day than any other. That taught me that the customer was not always right. I used this lesson later in life.

LESSON LEARNED
Working for the public is not always enjoyable!

Kimberly McBee

THE CLIENT I'LL NEVER FORGET

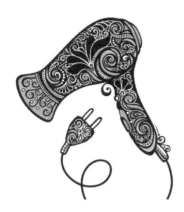

My head was down and I was sitting at the front desk of the salon. A man's voice said "Excuse me, what do you charge for a shampoo and set?"

I looked up and noticed a huge black man standing on the other side of the desk. He had bright blue contacts. He was startling to look at.

"Hello." I said with a jittery voice. "We charge nine dollars for a shampoo and set. Would you like to…" and before I could get another word out he said, "Can you take me now?" *YOU? Eh?"* he reiterated in his Canadian accent.

I thought, but didn't say… *What the hell,* but instead said, "I can take you right now, but I have never given a shampoo and set to a man before."

He chuckled and said, "I'll teach you." He was about six-feet-four and a huge build of a man. Not fat by any means, just big. I sat him down in my chair in front of my mirror and he took up the majority of it. I put my foot on the bar that moved the hydraulic chair down. I pushed it to the ground, using all my might, and it was already at the lowest it could go.

I began to see how it was—I was going to need to work on my tippy toes. I draped him and walked him back to a shampoo bowl. He sat in the chair, and then slid his butt down to the front of the chair so he could fit his thick neck into the neck holding portion of the bowl. I first rinsed his hair, and all sorts of colors came running out; first purple, then blue, then red, and pinks and greens, too. I asked about the psychedelic colors.

He said "I work for the circus. My wife and I work with the lions." He explained to me, still in his Canadian accent.

After shampooing for the first time, I asked if he would like me to condition his hair and he asked if I had oil. I told him that I had a moisturizer and he took me up on it.

Around that time in Eugene, we did not have many African Americans come into the salon. I did not have oil. But after doing Clint's hair that day, I bought some for the back bar. While the cream sat on his long black matted mass of hair, his wife walked in. She was six-feet-two, at least, and had long beautiful natural blonde hair, and wore fur boots to her thighs.

Amazon is the word I would use for this towering beautiful statuesque woman. She asked how long, and he told her about an hour. She nodded, without even looking once at me. I was staring at her with my mouth hanging open. She did not look human.

She looked like a fair skinned goddess. She left with a quick swivel of her boots.

Clint and I walked back to the chair that was lowered to the floor level. I was the only one at work that day. One employee was sick and others had taken the day off. I really liked working like this; it made it quite nice to talk to clients without others interrupting.

My class tutorial on how to do his hair began. He told me to show him my roller selection. I took out my beauty college rollers. I was embarrassed because they all have a #56 written in Sharpie on them, so he now knew I was pretty fresh out of school. But if it bothered him, he never let on.

He chose the biggest rollers I had in my Beauty College collection. I put in a sparkling gel-like styling aid. He seemed to like my choice. I applied the rollers the way he instructed and I placed this mountain of a man under the hood dryer. A great photo op!

I asked if he would like some water or coffee. He asked if we had tea. We have black tea.

"Black tea with two packets of sugar."

I poured his tea in a tiny tea cup like we serve the older women. I almost laughed when I handed the tiny tea cup over to his monster of a hand. He sipped his tea, drying for about three cups worth.

When the hood dryer shut off, I sat him back in my chair. I was behind the chair again, waiting for more instructions.

"Girl, just take them rollers out and run your finger through my hair and I'll pay you." As I removed the rollers we started a conversation that included questions about his job. Somehow he told me he was born in February, and so I told him I was too. He put his hand down the front of his shirt and grabbed out a huge amethyst stone made into a necklace. On any other person, it would look like a boulder, but on Clint it was just perfect. He told me, with a serious expression, "I also read minds."

WHAT? Oh my gosh—had he been reading my mind? Did he now know all my weird thoughts that I am having about him and his white Amazon Woman?

I took off the cape, and Clint stood up to his full height. I walked him to the desk cash register, and he paid his nine dollars and gave me my first tip of a ten dollar bill. Wow, he *must* have been reading my mind...

LESSON LEARNED
Beware of mind readers.

IT REALLY HAPPENED TO PAMELA

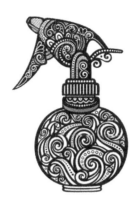

One day, an upbeat lady rolled in—in her wheelchair. She spoke energetically, before her wheels even had come to a stop. "What's shaken'?"

I looked up from the desk, smiled, and said, "Nothing. How can I help you?"

"Well, honey, I need a haircut." She was so happy she clearly made the people around her happy. Had I been in a bad mood, she would have changed it. I told her, I could take her if she could give me two seconds to finish a little book work.

Smiling, she told me, "Take your time. I have all the time in the world."

I like these types of people. They don't expect you to jump when they say they need something. I finished at the desk a few seconds later and wheeled Pamela back to my station, asking her, "What did you do to end up in the wheelchair?"

Gesturing towards her leg that was straight out

in front of her, supported by the wheelchair, she laughed and told me, "I stepped off the curb and got hit by the bus I was trying to catch."

"NO WAY?"

"Yes, I swear on my mother's grave that is what happened."

I did Pamela's hair and she loved it. She became one of my loyal clients, and even now I call her a friend—over 30 years later.

LESSON LEARNED

Stay on the curb until the bus comes to a complete stop.

ROOMMATE & LAUNDRY INCIDENTS

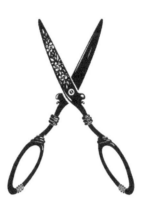

Wide Eyes and I had our differences. She was having boys over and drinking and partying. The last straw was when I came home from work and she was drinking alone on the hideaway bed that she had pulled out for a friend to sleep over, which never would fold up again. I guess that's what you get when you get hand-me-down furniture.

I figured she was going to keep doing foolish things. Maybe because of her sheltered life, she had decided to get crazy. Once, since we couldn't spend much on entertainment, I brought a guy I was dating home to watch some T.V. *The Late Show* with David Lettermen.

I had worked a long shift that day and fell asleep about twenty minutes into the show. I awoke to Wide Eyes and my date lying arm in arm, kissing on the floor next to me. I decided it was time for our roommate situation to come to an end—and to end it with the guy I was dating!

Wide Eyes saved me from forcing her out. *I learned not to fall asleep on a date, too.* A relative called, offering her an opportunity to move up north and start a new life. She did. I think it was to help her get back into the church. I didn't necessarily agree that her church was the best, but I did think that she needed something to calm her down.

Later I heard that she married a boy from her church and lived happily ever after.

This is when a friend from high school moved in—we lived comfortably in the apartment for a short time, but became *uncomfortable* (to say the least), when our landlord began walking into our apartment anytime she felt like it—like once when she barged in uninvited as my roommate was getting ready for work, and had on only her bra and panties. That did it. We decided to look for another place to live.

My roommate's older brother lived near us in a little house with his wife. They wanted to start a family and needed a bigger place. They asked if we would like to take over the rent and move into their little house. The rent was half of what we were paying, so we didn't even think twice.

We moved into the little house. It was located in front of a mill, still in Springfield. It had two bedrooms and one bathroom and the tiniest kitchen ever. But it was what we could afford at $180 a month. It probably should have been condemned—it was not insulated and we froze. I remember waking to frost on my down comforter. Thank God for blankets—and my brother's queen size waveless waterbed. I traded him for my king size waterbed. His was heated, which was great for me during those winter mornings under frost covered blankets. The wall heater worked really great, but it was so close that it singed my eyelashes while I slept.

We lived together in harmony because we both worked so much we never saw each other. I started dating more, which included seeing Mark. After being tied down in Beauty College with Logan (one controlling logger), I decided to be content with myself and find happiness in work, play, and dating.
Nothing too serious. We had parties and I was addicted to "PICTIONARY." I loved this game. We had friends over and played it for hours. I won a lot *and I didn't cheat.*

The little house had a place for a washer and dryer hook up, but we didn't have enough money to buy a set either, so we did the only thing we could; we saved our quarters for doing laundry.

One day I headed out with a car load of dirty clothes and had about three dollars in quarters. I thought... *okay, what do I really need to have clean?*

I went into the laundromat and put in enough quarters for one load of wash, carefully sorting my clothes to wash the essentials. When I went to dry them with my last quarters, the coin dispenser opened and popped out fourteen dollars in quarters. *Seriously, I thought I had won the lottery.* I was so excited. I will never forget it. I was able to do all my laundry, plus I had enough quarters to self-wash my Mustang. I drove home with my gold Mustang shining in the sun and the radio blasting Def Leppard's "Pour some Sugar On Me"... all the while feeling very lucky and content as I glanced back at my loads of CLEAN LAUNDRY!

The next time I headed to the laundromat, I had an incident after I put the first load in the car and ran back into the house to grab the next, leaving my pink Velcro purse in the front seat. After a couple of minutes, I got back to my car and my purse was gone. I saw some feet hopping over the fence in the back yard. I was too short to see over the fence and was so shocked that I didn't even try to run after the blue sneakers. Probably a smart call!

Well, there goes doing laundry, I thought. Then I remembered that my driver's license was in my purse, along with my first credit card I had ever gotten—a Montgomery Wards credit card, with my whopping ten percent discount for working there. (My first purchase was a VCR. I paid ten dollars a month to the one-hundred-ninety-nine dollar total for it. You would have thought I had spent one thousand; in my mind, I was being a big spender. That VCR lasted for 10 years.)

Anyway, back to the purse-napper. I cancelled my credit card and drove a few days without a driver's license until I could find time to go to the DMV. But the mill behind me saved me. I got a call from a man who told me they had found my purse and some items. He chuckled, which I thought was kind of odd.

I drove over to the mill and talked to the big, strong, older man and his crew. They were all snickering and giggling like a bunch of school girls. I could not figure out why they were acting like this. I walked up to talk with them. I could see my purse, so I thanked him, took it, and looked inside. My wallet was gone, but my driver's license was in my purse along with my lip gloss and a pack of juicy fruit gum and a couple of tampons. I thought... *Okay, is this why these grown men are acting like immature middle school boys?*

But no, the head man says, "Oh, here is something else that was in your purse, and he personally handed me my pack of birth control pills.

GREAT! Red faced, I thanked them all again, and went on my way. By the way, the purse was finally found on the back of a flat bed truck across town—and thankfully, my shop phone number was on my business card.

LESSON LEARNED
Some men never mature.

Kimberly McBee

WORKING FULL-TIME, PERMS PLUS

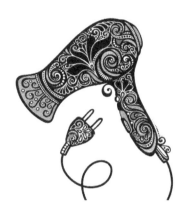

I worked Tuesday through Saturday, and still did not make enough, so I worked extra on my days off by going to people's homes. I gave perms for twenty dollars. I drove a lot with curlers and perm solution in the back of my gold Mustang hatchback. *Have perm will travel, or something like that!*

One job took me out to Lost Creek, way out in the country. A woman named Millie had gotten my name from another woman. She wanted a perm.

I arrived at her address and could not believe my eyes as I drove into the graveled driveway. The house looked like it should have been condemned. The siding was faded plywood. It had a few wooden chairs attached to the outside of the house. The house was a hanger for shovels and hoes, and even a wheelbarrow. The roof had dips where it was falling in. On the left side of the house three pit bulls stood barking at my car—and me! The dogs were in a kennel made of pig wire fence. I was not very comfortable getting out of my car. A woman came to the door and waved me in. I really wanted to rev up my Mustang and put it into reverse, do a one-eighty and get the hell out of there.

I needed the money, so I got out and walked up to the front door, forgetting my rollers. Millie told me to come on in. I walked into the house—evidently a hoarder's home. I could barely make my way through the dining area to the kitchen. My shoes stuck to the sticky floor, and I eyed Cheerios scattered all over the floor.

I told her I needed to grab my supplies, so I walked back out to the car. The barking dogs were at my back now. I should have gotten in the car to make a run for it. This was my second chance to escape, but I didn't take it. I grabbed the things I needed and headed back into the house filled with walls of boxes… and filth. For once, the perm solution might smell better than the house!

The kitchen was very small, but big enough for Millie to sit on a dining room chair, and for me to edge around it to work on her head. As I did the perm, she watched QVC on the sixteen inch T.V. It sat on her stained, previously white refrigerator.

Once I completed perming her hair, she was very grateful. She paid her twenty dollars; she set it on the table for me. I wanted to go as soon as possible, but some people are just lonely, and she was one, so I sat and visited with this freshly permed older woman while she served me some sort of tasteless tea. I can only hope that when I'm older, people will take the time with me that I have given to others over the years.

The stories... *just listen to their stories*. There is so much to hear and learn. Every eighty-year-old woman is a nineteen year old inside.

The oldest person I ever permed was one-hundred-three years old. This woman was lying in a bed when her daughter took me to her home. Her hair was in a braid to her knees and about as big around as my ring finger. It was very thin and white like snow. I don't think she wanted her hair cut, nor permed. In reality, I think she wanted to sleep and not wake up.

Her daughters and I worked together to get her seated in a chair. I cut her years of growth—and imagined the stories if her hair could talk. I made her short hair curly with the not so great smelling permanent wave solution. And when I was done, I encouraged her to look into a handheld mirror. I could tell by her expression that she did not recognize the person in the reflection. The look on her face was not a look of appreciation. She simply shrugged her shoulders, and casually took out her pipe, no joke, and she smoked some type of tobacco. It was like a scene from the old T.V. Show, "The Beverly Hillbillies."

The youngest I ever permed, was three. She was a cute little princess. Arielle was adopted from China and was the prettiest little doll. Her mother brought her into the salon when I worked in the mall. I sat her on a booster seat which made her look like she was seated on a throne—and she sat through the full perming experience, back straight, with better posture than any adult I had ever seen. I wondered about her. She acted as if she had come from royalty. Not much expression of any kind, even after I finished.

Her mother was very excited. She showed all kinds of expression. Don't get me wrong, but I think she was eager to show off her little China doll. I did not see love expressed towards the beautiful princess; it seemed more of an ownership to me. A reason to brag to her friends. I prayed this was not how it was for little Arielle.

I permed lots of men also. The one that I remember most was a father of four boys and one girl. He was the biggest Red Socks fan, I had ever met. He was masculine, and wore his curls with pride. His wife liked how I did his hair so well that she came to me for her hair. His daughter did also, and I still do her hair today.

LESSON LEARNED

The perm craze is over—and today, salons smell way better because of it.

Lessons Learned Behind the Chair

LOYALTY TO PAUL

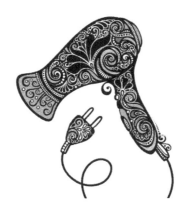

Remember Steve, Marks friend from the "Bleacher" story? His girlfriend, Connie, was a hairstylist. She wanted to work at a salon, so she came in one day when I was working and interviewed with Peru. She was hired and started the next day. (She filled the empty station Bonnie had left. You may remember the story about her being fired due to the missing money bag incident at Montgomery Wards Salon.)

Connie was a fabulous stylist. She shaved the sides of her head and wore leggings on the calves of her legs. She stood about five-feet-eight, and had an athletic build. She was no longer dating Steve, but had a new man in her life. Paul was his name. He seemed like a cool guy. Mark and I double dated with Connie and Paul a few times. He treated Connie with respect and you could tell he really cared for her. They moved in together. They met for lunch at the mall once in a while, so I noticed how they walked hand in hand. Even so, I felt at times, that she did not have the deep feeling that he felt for her.

As events would have it, Connie came to work in the afternoon one Tuesday. She was happier than I had seen her in a while. She was glowing! She said she was going to leave in an hour, so not to book her the whole afternoon. So I did as she asked and marked her books out. It seemed kind of odd, because Connie did nothing much, while I was working my fingers to the bone.

After being there for a total of forty-five minutes, a nice-looking guy came in and she left with this handsome man.

I had my break coming up for lunch and told Peru I would be back in thirty minutes. I walked behind Connie and the Good Looker. They walked, talked, and laughed with one another. We reached the glass doors to the outside. They proceeded on out and got into a black jeep. I had no idea who he was, but I thought Connie must be having an affair. I just kept thinking of her smitten live-in boyfriend, Paul.

Soon after, Connie came in to work. Paul had dropped her off. Once again, Connie walked right back out of the salon and jumped into the jeep again with Good Looker. I had, had it!

The phone rang at the front desk. I answered. It was a familiar voice. "Hey Kim, can I talk to Connie?

She has stepped out, Paul." I told him.

He was quiet. "Did she leave the store?" I hesitate and then replied "Yes, Paul."

I really liked Paul, and thought that if anyone was doing this to me, I would really want to not be made a fool of, so I told Paul that she left in a Jeep with someone. In the same breath, I told him we were looking for a roommate, because Mark and I had decided to move in together. We had found an apartment. (My roommate and I had realized that we had had enough of the friendship and roommate thing. She had started smoking cigarettes and the little house was starting to smell like an ashtray. Steve had started dating my roommate and he was over a lot of the time. Additionally, my roommate's sister, who had gotten out of the military, had practically moved in and was sleeping on our couch—and for lack of a better word, she was not very honorable as a roommate.)

Mark was staying over a lot and he wanted out where he lived. We had found a nice two bedroom, two baths, and on the bottom floor. Time to play house. We moved in and found that the family who lived above us was *not* drug dealers, they were bow hunters. Their daughter loved her roller-skates, and skated day *and some nights* on the floor above us... *but oh well!* There was an in-ground pool with no heater—and in Oregon this was not ideal... *but again... oh well!*

Paul called a few days later, and he moved in with Mark and me in our new apartment. It all worked out great, and it was so exciting to play house. We purchased a used clothes dryer for the apartment right after we moved in. An interesting story resulted, because while doing a load, it caught on fire. That was another new challenge—but Mark put it out without hesitation.
Everyone survived.

LESSON LEARNED
Don't mess around in relationships—you might get caught.

BANDIT

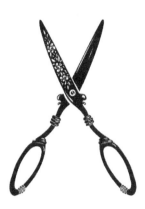

Many clients had told me not to get a dog in an apartment. They especially advised me to *definitely not* get a puppy. But sometimes I just wanted to learn the hard way.

It was Mark's birthday. I watched the classified ads and found two different *puppy* options. The first was an ad for a litter of Beagles, one month old. The second was for six-week-old Schnauzers.

I called and made an appointment to go and see the Schnauzers. Walking up to the door of the owner's home all I heard was *yap, yap, yap.* I thought before the door ever opened... *I am going to go with a beagle.*

I went ahead and walked into the Schnauzer house that looked like a person could eat off the floor. They must not work—just clean house all day. It was spotless, but I was not buying a house, but a dog and these would not stop barking! I was done with my visit in minutes. I told the woman that I lived in an apartment and needed a quieter dog. *Thanks, but no thanks.*

I went to the next appointment to see the lady with the Beagle puppies. I pulled into the driveway and admired the well kept yard full of flowers and perfectly trimmed grass. I walked to the door and knocked. Nothing. *I mean, no barking.* I was pleasantly surprised.

The woman came to the door. She reminded me of a woman I played softball with. Short, clean cut hair, and almost masculine features. She greeted me with a smile.

"Hello," I said, and she told me to come on in. Her partner was sitting on the couch, and she called the two dogs over who were the mother and father. These dogs were tricolored and show quality. Then she put them in the back room and showed me the four baby Beagles in the fluffy cream colored dog bed. It was love at first sight. I chose the medium-sized one who was snugly. I asked if I could make payments and they agreed. I could not wait to take Bandit home, but I had to wait two weeks, so I paid my down payment and left, feeling excited and satisfied with this puppy.

Two weeks later, I tied a red ribbon around the puppy's neck and waited for Mark to come home to see the big surprise for his birthday. I would not say Mark was excited, but after awhile Bandit grew on him. Maybe like a fungus. (If you ever saw "Marley and Me," you get the picture of how destructive Bandit became.)

We named him Bandit due to the fact that he

had a diamond on his back and a black "mask" around his eyes like thick eyeliner. We left him in our apartment while we worked. He ripped Mark's favorite pillow in half and I thought Mark was going to cry. I laughed it off until the next day when he did the same to my pillow. I had had that bed pillow since I was a child. I did cry. Every time we came through the door at home, something else was being torn to pieces. He even went after the carpet! He tore a hole so big in it; we could set our up-right vacuum inside it.

Easter, Paul brought home a chocolate solid chocolate Easter bunny and Bandit ate it while we were working. I know, I know chocolate is not good for dogs, but he did it, not me. After Bandit had eaten it, I came home to Mark and Paul sitting on our couch watching Bandit run laps around and around and around for hours in the apartment. He collapsed, and slept, I swear, for two days. Bandit was our first experience with taking care of something together. Hmm...

LESSON LEARNED
Dogs are a pain, but lovable.

Kimberly McBee

NAKED IN MORE WAYS THAN ONE

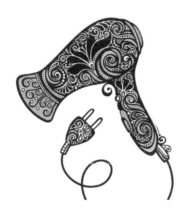

Roommates, roommates, roommates! I never wanted to introduce Mary to any other guy ever since I had played matchmaker with the logger who had cheated on her—back when we were in Beauty College.

It went down something like this: Mary had gone over one evening to see Randy, who was the logger who worked with Logan, my "limousine" logger boyfriend.

The door was locked, so she thought she would sneak into the window and surprise him. She did, but the surprise was on Mary. There was another woman in bed with her boyfriend, and she was not wearing a stitch of clothing. But neither was he.

Fast and with force Mary pulled the blankets off them. Randy awoke, very startled, and grabbed the blanket and covered himself. Mary pulled the naked woman from the bed by her hair. Randy laughed, once he realized what was happening, which only made the situation worse.

Mary yelled and cursed loud enough for Randy's brother to wake up. His brother, in his tighty whiteys, picked Mary up and carried her out the door. She fought and clawed her way, wanting to kill the stripper in Randy's bed. I decided after that fiasco; *no more introducing friends to friends.*

My commitment was short-lived, because Paul, our roommate, was single (after Connie cheated on him)—and he was a little leery of getting involved with anyone. Even so, he asked me if I knew anyone that he could take to the Lane County Fair, so we could all go together. I told him I did not have the best experience in playing Cupid.

I can give it a try, I thought. I went ahead and sat a picture and phone number down on the counter in our kitchen of our apartment—Mary. I told him it was up to him to initiate the meeting.

Mark saw the picture and he said "SHE IS A STONE FOX!" I had never heard this before and never have since. Yes, this was my dork boyfriend.

Within minutes of seeing her picture, Paul called Mary. She came to the fair with us, along with another couple who were friends from California.

Long story short, Mary and Paul became inseparable. One day when Paul came home from the river, I asked what they had been up to and he told me that they had gone to the river and sunbathed in the nude. "WHAT?"

I hadn't known, but Paul had been raised as a nudist. He had talked Mary into going topless. She wore a thong. They had fun in the sun—and didn't get too many tan lines. I was sort of jealous, but

could never bring myself to rip off my clothes in front of people. They are still nudists—and have two boys, and are living happily ever-after in Florida.
Miss you two!

LESSON LEARNED
With some friends you can pick up right where you left off—no matter the distance or years apart.

Kimberly McBee

ASKING FOR MY HAND

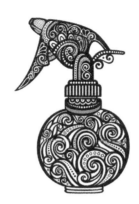

It was the end of a long work week, and I came home to the carpet-eaten apartment. I was exhausted. It was Friday, and I had arranged for Saturday off. Mark and I were excited to take off to go camping.

Camping was a great weekend get away, and we always took "Bandit the Destroyer." He was a loving dog. It wasn't his fault; we should have never gotten a dog while living in an apartment and working all day. He was just bored.

Mark got home and laid down next to me on the bed. I was motionless, fully dressed with my feet still on the floor. He plopped next to me, our heads next to each other. We were supposed to be packing. He looked like I felt, totally exhausted. "Do you want to go?" he asked.

"I do," I said, "But I don't want to move. I want to go to sleep."

"So we are staying home?" he asked.

"YES!" I said, not really wanting to, but my eyes and body were working against me. I knew Mark's job was very labor intensive, as was mine. Being a hair stylist is not thought of as labor intensive and physical, but I was on my feet all day, sometimes twelve hours straight. This profession can be emotionally exhausting, too, dealing with people's vanity. Different personalities force stylists to become chameleons to suit each person in the chair. It's a rewarding job, but hard work, nonetheless.

Back to me lying on the bed, my sore feet on the floor. I couldn't help myself; I started to fall asleep in the same position. I heard Mark get up. He changed into shorts, or what he calls, getting comfy. He laid back on the bed in the same position that I was in. Both our heads were together, almost touching. He said "I was going to do this while we were camping, but since we are not going..."

He hesitated, and I started to realize he was talking and I needed to listen and stop drifting off. "Will you marry me?"

Okay, I'm awake now! I said nothing for a second or two, and then took in the moment. Romantic, not so much, but I loved that he had planned to ask me while we were camping out in the woods. He handed me a ring that he had picked out by himself. I put it on and shortly after we were both asleep in the same positions—with me still fully dressed.

LESSON LEARNED
Romance is all in the eye of the beholder.

TEARS OF DISTRESS

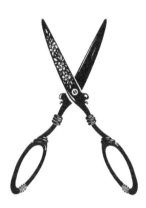

It was Thursday and I only had two more days left of my work week. A woman walked in almost in tears. She told me she came from what I called, the fancy "Paris Hair Salon" in the upstairs of the mall. (Remember, it is the one from an earlier story, the salon where the manager would not let us in for a tour—students from the Beauty College.)

Anyway, this poor woman, Val, had asked for her hair to be colored darker, but they had turned it pitch black. I consoled her and sat with her in the tiny waiting area. I convinced her I could help and change her Witchy look. Val had pretty dark eyes and a snow white look to her fair skin.

We used my precut foils—not to wrap leftovers or steak, but to highlight her hair. After this effectively removed the black, she loved the chocolate brown with auburn highlights that reflected back at her from the mirror.

I never understood salons that charged so much and thought they were so much better. They intimidated clients, so they rarely asked for their money back in such places, because they are too embarrassed. I sympathize, because she spent lots of her hard earned money—and came out a disaster. Yes, people do pay as much as two-hundred-fifty dollars to look like count Dracula's bride!

The next over-the-top color correction I did was a middle-aged working woman who came in with what I presumed was her attempt to bleach her full head of hair blonde, but instead she got the brassy, trailer trash blonde that was in dire need of hydration. It reminded me of Beauty College and my first model experience. Not good!

I treated her with kindness and told her a conditioning treatment was where we would start. I asked how long she had been coloring her own hair, and she replied that she just gotten it done at, you guessed it, "Paris Salon!" I asked her who had done this and she gave me the name of a stylist. It sounded familiar.

Yes, it was the same as the correction I had done on the previous day. I marked my full day out; since it was a walk-in salon I could do this. I conditioned her hair and talked to her about how we could take her blonder and tone it, or go with a darker shade that would be more complementary to her skin tone.

She told me, "Do anything, as long as it doesn't look like this."

I said, "Giving a stylist free rein to do whatever she wants, may be part of your problem—

something outlandish like this is the result."

I taught her how to be her own advocate during the hair consultation. "Make sure you are with a stylist who listens—and don't trust that you will love whatever they do." I went on to encourage a confident attitude. "You should have some sort of an idea and be able to explain what you want, before you ever walk into the salon—or at least know your stylist can be trusted. Tastes and skills vary with each stylist. She seemed a little on the conservative side, so I asked lots of questions to determine what she wanted.

Do you work from home? Are you able to come in regularly for color touch up maintenance?

She told me that she worked outside the home and time is limited. She said that she could make time for a six-week maintenance plan to color and hide her gray hair.

We visited while the conditioner was soaking into her gold, almost slimy hair. I enjoyed her, a really great lady. I learned that she had two boys; both adopted both from the U.S. They were not from the same biological parents.

As a stylist, I've always felt that it's good to know who my client's are as people, and then fit their style to what they want everyone else to see. Her build was medium size, and she had a lot of hair, and did not want to look like a glimmering ball of sunshine.

After rinsing the conditioning goodness from her hair, I placed her under a dryer with a filling agent. The hair, when bleaching is done to that extent, is so porous that it will not hold hair color unless filled.

We talked more while she was under the hooded dryer. I enjoyed taking lots of time to show her color swatches, and suggested a gorgeous shade of reddish brown natural—with attitude! She liked it. I laughed and told her, "It will make your blue eyes stand out and your husband will think he is sleeping with another woman. She smiled; took my advice.

We applied the reddish brown color to her dry hair and I threw in a few highlights. I waited the needed time, giving a gentle shampoo, conditioning again; this time with a fade prevention conditioner. After three hours, we dried and styled her beautiful new look. I cut it into a shorter layered look—she looked sporty. She hugged me while paying for her service, and rescheduled for her next hair experience. A happy new client!

I wanted to go straight up the escalator to the "Paris Salon, and slap the stylist for turning this poor woman into a freak. *But I guessed that would not make me look too professional.*

Later that day, I did call the salon and ask for the manager. I told her about the two women that had come into my salon. Do you know what she said in her snooty voice? "Oh, is that right?" She did not care one bit about the less than professional outcome for the two women.

I wondered later if she might have been the stylist who had done their hair. I never did get her name. *OOPS!*

LESSON LEARNED
If you think your shit doesn't stink, you're wrong!

Lessons Learned Behind the Chair

Kimberly McBee

NINE-TO-FIVE BURNOUT

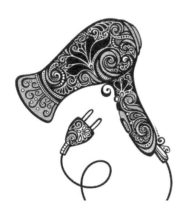

Working with a new client each appointment can get tiring beyond words. They sometimes want things they cannot have due to not enough hair or the right type of hair. *Or they may want to look like the model in the magazine.* (Don't we all!) Some do not look at the hair style, but it's the image they really want.

I had a young woman come to me, and she tilted her head at a ninety degree angle and held it there, telling me she wanted her hair to stay like that. The entire appointment time, I was thinking to myself... *Crazy, whacko! Please Calgon take me away*—like the old commercial that showed a contented woman soaking in a tub full of white fluffy bubbles. Yes!

I realized I needed a change; I was feeling burnt out. A family need presented itself, and I had an idea. Mark's grandmother had had a stroke. I knew she was in a nursing home and did not want to be there. I couldn't blame her. She had always been an active, outdoorsy-type of woman. (Meaning, she wanted to be out with the men rather than in the house doing domestic chores.) I could relate, I would much rather be mowing the lawn than cleaning a bathroom or kitchen any day.

Mark's aunt, from California, was trying to get her out of the nursing home and hire a full time nurse, but that was not an easy task. I talked with Mark and suggested that we do it.

I thought that we could move out of the apartment that we shared with Paul and help his grandmother in her home. Her daughter, Aunt June, had remodeled her cute little one bedroom house near the lake, making it wheelchair accessible. It was clean, and it had nice blue carpet and white linoleum with little dainty blue flowers, all new appliances—and by making the most of Grandma's antique furnishings, it was adorable on the inside. Perfect for his grandmother to spend her last days if she had the support she needed.

So, I had this brilliant idea, I was still not making a lot of money, so if Aunt June paid us, and I learned the caretaking skills needed, she could save on the expense of a full time nurse. We could move in with Grandma Dorothy and take care of her. Aunt June and her husband liked this idea, too.

Mark and I knew Paul was moving in with Mary, and the rent at our apartment was going up another hundred dollars a month, so it was a win-win for everyone. I could also get off my feet day-in and day-out, and keep my sanity. I did not want to end up smacking someone with a blow dryer, and getting sued!

We moved into Grandma's little 720 square foot "shack" as she called it. It was in a small town about fifteen minutes from my job. If she started getting better, I planned to go back to work part time. Next, we brought Grandma Dorothy home, and put a hospital bed in the front room. She was paralyzed on one side of her body and could not speak. She was still with it though, and I could tell she was glad we were there.

She loved sports, so she and Mark would watch basketball together. Mark did all the yelling for her. I wanted to give her a foam block or something to throw at the screen. It was exciting and fun for her—and us.

A nurse came in and taught me how to change her and move her from side to side with blankets, using my upper body strength. It really is a special technique, and if not done right, it can put caretakers in a chiropractor's office.

Unfortunately, she hated Bandit. She never spoke, but when he would get into her flower beds, then she would use her words—yell, was more like it. Clear as a bell, she would say, "NO DOG!"

I was on the phone with Aunt June telling her the move went well. It was a relief for her and she had no worries. Over the phone, she heard the,
"NO DOG!"

June asked, "Who was that?"

"That was your mother." I said "She is not a fan of Bandit, our dog."

You keep that dog around," she said, "if it will keep her talking."

A month went by, and Mark and I decided to

take an evening off and go out with friends. It was like having a child. We got a sitter. We hired one of the caregivers that came in once in a while when I went grocery shopping and out to do errands.

After a fun evening of catching up with Mary and Paul, and night club dancing, we found ourselves home by midnight. The caregiver said everything had gone well. We paid her and she was on her way. Dorothy was sound asleep. So we headed to bed.

Two hours later I got up to check on her and she had thrown her blanket on the ground and taken off all her clothes. *How in the hell did she manage that?* So... I turned on a side table lamp and re-dressed her. I checked her bedding and tucked her in again. Snug as a bug in a rug.

I went to the restroom and came in to turn off the light. There on the floor was the blanket—again! She was tugging at her clothes. I didn't think she was hot. She didn't even seem awake.

I repeated the process of tucking her in and turned off the light and told her I'd see her in the morning.

When I awoke at four, she had done it all again.

Poor soul. She was done. She seemed to just want life to be over. I think that she had come home to say goodbye.

I gently told her, "Grandma Dorothy, you are going to freeze to death." I changed her bedding and night clothes, so she was dry and fresh.

I thought she was sound asleep when I went to bed. Not! She did it again as soon as I went to bed. Sneaky.

The following morning I woke up, pushed the button for the coffee and stepped into the front room. There she was, just like the day she was born. I rushed to get her covered before her grandson came out. She was asleep—and I got her covered with blankets.

After Mark left for work, I struggled to get her dressed once again. I noticed her breathing was raspy. Right away, I called and talked with the nurse who was coming that day. She told me to call 911. I did.

About that time, my sister drove into my driveway, and when I opened the door Bandit got out. He did that a lot. I greeted my sister and her two kids. "Kathy, this is not a good time!" Before she could leave, the ambulance was there to pick up Dorothy. I told the ambulance driver I would follow them. They took her to the local hospital.

I caught Bandit with the help of my sister and her kids. I called my father and mother-in-law, and Aunt June to tell them what was going on. Then I drove to the hospital.

She had pneumonia. She stayed in the hospital resting comfortably. She was in good hands. The next morning I got the call that she had passed away. We had no idea she would go so fast. I was thankful she got to come home, to her little shack, and to spend time with her grandson. After her stroke, she did not want to live like that—and I know she is in a better place.

LESSON LEARNED
Getting old is not for wimps!

BACK BEHIND THE CHAIR— TO ACTION HAIR

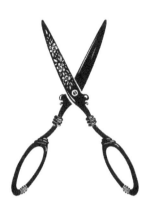

Bonnie (remember, she is the one with the big band hair who was fired for the lost cash bag at the Montomery Wards salon) called me one day when I had had enough at the little outdated salon I worked in. "What's up, Kim?"

"I'm okay, how are you doing?" I replied. She was working at another salon on the west side of town, for a private owner. She asked me the right things at the right time.

She said, "The salon I'm working in is awesome, and they have an empty station. I told them about you and how you need to get out of Montgomery Wards. Are you still doing the payroll and not getting paid for it?"

"Yes, I am." I whispered, since I was talking on the Montgomery Ward's Salon telephone.

"I'm going to tell the owner, Rose that you are

coming in on Monday to check out the salon and to meet her." She will be excited to meet you. Bonnie was supposedly asking me—but clearly, she was not taking no for an answer.

On Monday morning, I dressed professionally for my meeting. I showed up at 10:00 a.m. I could see Bonnie in the window, and she greeted me with a smile. This shop was also closer, which was important since we had bought Grandma Dorothy's house from the family after she passed. We would be there for a while.

As I walked toward the front door of the salon, I loved that there was a huge window in the front and a glass door which meant sunlight. I had been in a cube with no natural light for long enough.

I walked in with high hopes. My hope dwindled down a bit when I entered. The salon had six stations and three shampoo bowls and a back room with about six hood dryer chairs. This was bigger, yes, with the best part being the huge window, but little else.

I looked around and saw there was a big break room and a one stool bathroom. The front desk was fake wood and white Formica. The shop was long and deep and narrow. Three stations on one side had one long mirror in front of them. The walls were the same orange as the Wards salon. The chairs were brown and the shampoo bowls had a reclining chocolate brown chair. So 70s!

Above Rose's station, she was growing a jungle. A flowering plant started at her station table top and wrapped up around her mirror. I was glad to see the salon was clean.

Way in the back stood a torture chamber from the 1920s and 30s. This was an antique perming machine that was not used. It was just for show. Back in the day, these types of perm machines attached a clients perm rods to it. I had heard there were tons of chemical burns back then. I even had a client who had used such a thing.

Her name was Ester, and she was an award winning beautician back in the day. She said she took home the papers after they used them for the perm and put them in the fireplace and burned them and they made beautiful colors. I always wondered... *What was that doing to her lungs?*

Rose, the owner, walked in. Rose had worked in a salon since she was a teen. Rose was a large woman, in her fifties. She had faded red hair. It looked like she could not commit to the red. She walked over to me and I noticed she was pigeon toed. She was wearing polyester. My mother always wore polyester too, well past its popularity. I guess it's an era thing.

I introduced myself and Rose walked me into the back room. It served as both a break room and chemical dispensary. I was wearing the same dress I got for graduation from Beauty College. When I bought it, I had never seen a dress quite this color. It was a pretty sky blue and buttoned down the front. It had a blousy top and was form fitting through the bottom. Size seven—I can only wish for that size to work for me today.

Rose seemed nice enough. We talked about which days I was available. I told her I always worked one night a week, and Tuesday through

Saturday, having Sunday's and Monday's off. This is a normal stylist schedule. Some days I worked, nine to nine, and got time to pee for good behavior.

She agreed with my schedule preference, since she closed on those days. I told her I didn't know how many clients would follow. I had told people I might be making a move and they were excited for me. I asked the prices she charged, and shared what I had been charging and she laughed. "You are giving your services away," she said.

She handed me the price list and it was almost double, which meant more take home pay for me. I told her I would need to be guaranteed eight hundred a month because that was what I was making over at the mall. She said I would receive fifty percent in commission or minimum wage, whichever was higher. The minimum wage, then, was around $3.75 an hour, and the state was talking about raising it. I told her that was great, but I have to be guaranteed $400 take home a paycheck or $800 a month. Before I left the shop, Rose made her decision. I was to start in two weeks. This gave me enough time to put in my two week notice and tell clients of my change in location. After four years at the mall, I was making a move.

LESSON LEARNED
Making a decision to move takes you on a new path.

OUR WEDDING

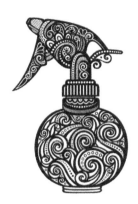

In May, 1989, our wedding date was set for the 20th. I was about to marry my best friend. I wanted an outdoor wedding, my mother wanted a church wedding, and Mark did not care, he just wanted it over!

We married in a tiny country church close to where I grew up. Short and sweet was a request from my tall, dark, and handsome soon to be husband.

The reception was in the church basement with cake, punch, nuts and mints. Old school, I know, but that is what my mother had pictured for me. At least I got an outdoor receiving line—and the day was gorgeous.

I paid $125.00 for my wedding dress out of the JC Penny's Catalog. It looked like Snow White's dress if she was to get married—lacey, big and fluffy. The wedding decorations were done by my mother—her floral school arrangements. A friend from high school, did my bouquet; it was roses and orchids and absolutely beautiful.

My colors were royal blue and fuchsia. (Remember, it was the 80s!) The bridesmaids all wore royal blue with fuchsia accents in the flowers. I wore white, of course, and I forced my poor, sweet Mark to wear white tails. (Don't ask me why, but it was one thing that I really wanted control over.) Oh boy, I hear about it even today—sorry honey. He was a good sport, and in my defense, he only had to wear it for a short period of time. Good or bad, the pictures last forever—to be seen by family and friends for posterity.

A friend did our photography, as we poked cake in each others' faces. Then we had a lovely toast with sparkling apple cider. (I wish it could have been champagne, but we were in church, remember?) We then went back upstairs, and spent lots of time saying "cheese." When all the pictures were taken, we went back down to enjoy the people at the reception, only to find cleanup being done and everyone gone. We had missed it all.

LESSON LEARNED

Take wedding pictures before the wedding or you miss your own party.

HONEYMOON

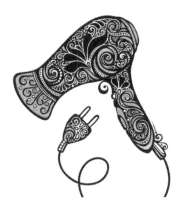

While in the receiving line at the wedding, Mark's Aunt June and her husband Dean came through and congratulated us. They hugged us, and then gave us the kindest gift I have ever received. An all expense paid trip to Hawaii—including the hotel and the airfare.

Before receiving this kind gift, our plan was to drive to San Francisco with eight hundred dollars we had saved—we figured when the money ran out we would come home.

June and Dean had even planned our trip for us, and we were to leave the next day. "Sneaky they were," as Yoda would say.

Mark had never been to the island and neither had I. Fun memories came from watching all the tourists run for cover when Hawaii dosed us with its daily rain sprinkles. Hell, we are from Oregon! We did not run; we just loved the warm, sweet rain on our skin.

Mark and I rented a convertible and drove around the island, and for the first time saw how pineapple was grown—not in trees like I had always thought. I was twenty-two and so was Mark. *I guess we didn't know everything!*

We visited Pearl Harbor and met a man who had been on the Arizona the day they were bombed. He was blown off the battleship, so interesting and sad at the same time to get to hear his personal story.

We took an excursion on the water (booze cruise), and found out that I get sea sick. Mark had fun, me… not so much.

Advice for new travelers: Don't try to do too much, enjoy yourself and don't take too many excursions. We discovered it is almost more fun to buy a six pack and sit on the beach. (Our last honeymoon night.)

LESSON LEARNED
Simple is quite nice.

NEW JOB, FRESH PATH

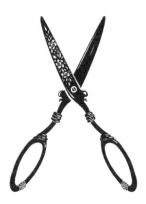

Starting a new job is always a chore. Even with it being the same type of job I was trained for, I was in a different place and getting used to unfamiliar things.

My new station was on the north wall instead of the east wall. I noticed Bonnie was busy with clients and happy as ever at this salon. I was undecided. It was quieter, so different from being in a busy mall with people walking in constantly—but I focused on the one thing I loved—the big window—it was a plus.

Tracy was one of the stylists. She was in her early twenties, and she had come from the "Paris Salon." (Maybe she had been the one to do the color fiascos!) She thought her shit did not stink. I was not too impressed. Don't get me wrong, she was a good stylist, but her attitude was too stuck up for my taste. She was very choosy about the clients who got to sit in her chair. She was married and pregnant with her first child. I was glad to know she was taking maternity leave soon.

And then there was Melanie. She was a stylist with, I believe, the early stages of dementia. She had a mousy look and dressed from Goodwill. Not much style, but I learned later she was a single woman who was just trying to make it after her husband left her. She was in her mid-fifties, the same age as Rose, my new boss.

My first client in the new job had never been to this salon. I liked that, because she had no expectations from previous experiences with stylists here. I greeted her at the front waiting area with the huge window. I said "Hello, I understand you have never been in before…"

She smiled, "Yes, that's right."

I asked, "What is your name?"

She told me, "Patricia." We chatted and looked at the pictures she had brought in from different magazines. I have learned through the years that most women will pick the same haircut, just slightly different on how it looks on three or more models.

I told her it was a great choice and would look great on her face shape. I found out while walking her back to my station that a client I did regularly had referred her to me. This was the first person I brought into my new job by referral. This impressed Rose. I was pretty excited to show off my skills.

Patricia and I talked about color. I talked her into doing it that day. *Why not?* I had the time. She had always been dishwater blonde. When Patricia left, she wore honey blonde highlights and she was looking short, sassy and sexy. Just what she asked for.

Tracy, who thought she knew everything, then started asking me questions. Sometimes if you come off your high horse you learn some things.

LESSON LEARNED
Change is a good thing.

Kimberly McBee

Lessons Learned Behind the Chair

REMEMBERING BILLIE

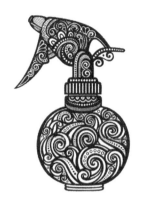

One sunny day, a very pregnant, very exhausted, beautiful young woman walked in and was standing at the front desk. I walked over and she spoke in such a high volume you could have heard her in the next room. Her accent was none I had heard before. I couldn't understand her, and thought maybe it was German or Russian?

I took her to my chair and she was glad to get the weight off her swollen feet. Billie was her name. She was thin, except for her ginormous belly. It was hotter than Hades outside and I felt so sorry for my new client and soon-to-be friend. The heat was making her miserable. Her baby was ready to show his face any day.

All she said was, "SHORT!" I cut her hair short and cooled her with a nice cooler rinse at the shampoo bowl, and she became a loyal client for a very long time.

Billie had her baby and I gave him his first haircut after his first birthday. He sat in the chair as proud as he told me about his "Thomas the Train" knowledge. He banged his train on the hand bar. He lifted his hand and hit me so hard in the head that I thought I was going to black out. I excused myself and walked back to the back break room.

The room was spinning. I nearly got a concussion from a one year old! Are you kidding me? I have played sports all my life and even played on coed teams. But I ended up with a slight concussion from a toddler banging a "Thomas the Train" toy.

After getting a drink of water, I put on a smile and returned to cut Thomas's hair. I don't remember doing it!

LESSON LEARNED
I don't know my accents very well. Billie was from Austria.

T.M.I.

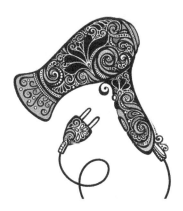

Have you ever been told just "**T**oo **M**uch **I**nformation?" Well, I had Marguerite in my chair and as I stood behind it, this seventy-year-old woman was telling me all about her sex life with her husband. I wanted to stuff cotton in my ears. Don't get me wrong, I'm not a prude. In fact, almost the opposite, but this was putting unwanted pictures in my head.

In great detail, Marguerite went on about her new, sexy negligee she had just bought. Apparently it was a soft pink and the nipples were cut out with crotchless undies to boot. "Lovely!" I said.
Thinking... *What the hell am I saying?*

She was smiling a Cheshire cat grin, just like someone that had just smoked a bowl and had a permagrin grin on her face. She was wearing bright red lipstick, with some stuck on her two front teeth. She continued to tell, exposing me to what excited Fred, her husband, and I thought I was going to get sick. This had to have been the longest hair appointment in history. I love stories people have to tell, but these sex life visuals were too strong for my taste.

I have learned not to get into politics or religion, and have added this to my list—not to get into hearing about the sex lives of women over seventy, especially when they tell too much detailed information!

One woman told me she had lost all her hair on her legs and under her arms, but was most excited to tell me that she had also lost all of her hair down under. She was not talking about Australia.

LESSON LEARNED
Fred knows how to please his lady.

COUPONS AND SALES

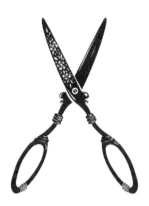

Rose loved to put perms on sale, even though we had plenty of perm clients all the time. I told her we should advertise something else, like color, but she wanted to do more perms. In the huge window, it read: $30 PERMS. Walk-ins Welcome.
She might as well have said: Come on in, you cheap jerks who expect everything for nothing!

My bad experience was with a lady of middle age and medium length hair. I permed her hair and she was so happy. She left after paying her $30. Great, I had not made the money I had wanted, but she was happy. Two and one half hours of work— and I got fifty percent. Then, divided by two, I got about $3.75 an hour. Rose paid $5 for the perm solution so she gained $10. After taxes... you understand. We both got screwed.

This particular "coupon special" lady came back the next day. She didn't like her perm. It looked just as it had the day before when she loved it. Now she wanted *all* her money back.

I wanted Peru as a boss again, because she stood up for what was right. Not Rose. She stood there listening to this lady's complaint, not saying a word. She just listened in silence. I saw her nod her head once in a while. Then Rose gave her cash back, and the lady walked out with a smirky look on her face—because she had just gotten away with it.

"Peru, where are you?" Peru would have yelled and called her a thief. I told myself that day, that if I ever owned my own salon, I would not give back money unless there was something truly wrong. I would stand up for my employees, like Peru had done for me.

LESSON LEARNED
Don't give your work away; the gesture can come back and bite you in the butt!

WELCOME WAGON

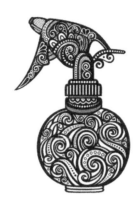

As I said in the last story, my boss liked to give our work away, but Welcome Wagon was an okay way to advertise and gain new people that had just moved to the area. The Welcome Wagon was a service to new people moving into our city and the nearby areas. We offered a free haircut from our salon, that Welcome Wagon gave out when they met the new arrivals to our area. It was a crap shoot which one of us would get these people walking in with their invitation to our salon for their freebie.

One day a woman came in, with a Welcome Wagon invite, and I was the only one in-between clients. She was well dressed and had a kind face. I greeted her at the front desk and we both said hello at the same time. After that, we laughed at the same time after that. I knew then we were a good match.

I directed her back to the chair. Behind the chair

I consulted with Darlene and she listened to my suggestions. I recommended a razor cut. (This is where you cut the hair with a straight or feather razor. It's a disposable blade, so you cannot cut yourself with these blades, or the client.) It's a little safer for your victim and your phalanges. Definition for phalanges (fingers.) Darlene liked the razor-cut idea and we headed to the shampoo bowl.

My job may seem repetitious. It is not. You have a new person in your chair every hour or two. It can be fun, rewarding and sometimes crazy. Darlene enjoyed the shampoo—and I took my time and helped her feel and experience my expertise.

I had decided to move to a new salon soon. I needed to let her know, so if she wanted to follow me she could. So I secretly told her.

I still feel bad about taking a client Rose had gotten through advertising through Welcome Wagon. But I made Rose lots of money by bringing in most of the clients from my last salon location. So, I guess I did not need to feel that bad.

Darlene still comes to me today. Love her...

LESSON LEARNED
Clients that have loyalty are the best!

COLLEAGUES

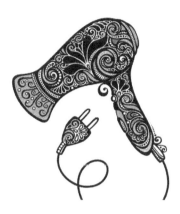

Mary, my friend, was coming to work with me at Rose's salon—and I loved it. She was a hard worker. Jo, her buddy from school was fifty-some years old with kids our age. Jo came in to interview and she was hired the same time as Mary. I did not think Rose was making a wise decision by hiring them at the same time. I was concerned about us all staying busy. There may not be enough clients to go around, but apparently Mary had made it an all or nothing deal.

They had graduated together, after me, and they had both worked at the mall, but in a different salon than me. They were together all the time. They had some loyal clients, but not enough to keep them busy all the time.

Mary was my age, but maybe one year older. She was now engaged to Paul, our old roomie. Jo seemed to pick up lots of middle-aged business people—teachers, nurses, and store clerks. Mary collected men who chose a lot of clipper cuts "barbarism."

Each one of us excelled in our special cuts and chemical talents. Now Bonnie excelled in men, but now I'm not talking about work. She shared about dating a different man every night.

I was not the only one she told her wild stories. She loved entertaining her clients with her stories of meeting some guy at a bar and taking him home, or meeting some man in a dance club and going back to his place. She worried me. I thought for sure she would come to work one day and tell me she had some untreatable venereal disease. I never heard.

She started dating one of the football players from the local university. She fell hard for him. He was a well built, black tight end. Yes, his tight end looked good to me. I don't know if he knew what he was getting into with wild Bonnie.

One day at work, she was backcombing this elderly lady's hair. She was giving her a pretty full-blown description of sleeping with this well built college football player.

As she and her elderly client were giggling, in walks a police officer fully dressed in his blue uniform. At the same time, Rose came out of the break room where she was most of the time. (Since she had so many stylists on the floor, she did not need to work behind her chair as often. This was good because she was loosing her touch in my opinion).

My patron and I, and all the other patrons in the shop, watched the drama unfold as the police asked, "Are you Bonnie?" She started to reply. Yes, but before she could make up a response he was handcuffing her from the back. She was laughing with her girlish-like giggle.

Bonnie was led out the door. None of us knew what she had been arrested for—and Rose being Rose, she walked over like nothing had happened, and finished Bonnie's back combing. The shop was so morgue quiet you could hear a bobbie pin hit the floor.

LESSON LEARNED
Don't do the crime if you can't do the time!

Kimberly McBee

LEAVE THE BABY AT HOME

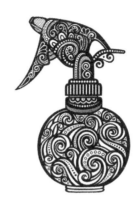

An ongoing dilemma for women is how they can juggle all their roles. Like my coworker, Tracy, who came back to work at Rose's Action Salon after having her baby boy. She had a hard time returning to work, because that meant she would have to pump to provide her milk for the little babe.

It's just my opinion, but I feel bad for women who have to pump with a machine, like a cow milking machine. She could not handle it, so once her cute little bundle of joy was old enough to be put in a play pen she brought that darn play pen into the shop. Who gets to bring their children with them to work?

TRACY, she was a favorite for sure. Don't get me wrong, the little guy was cute. He was especially cute when sleeping. Nap time was my favorite!
He pretty much yelled for his mother the whole time she was working. Oh, Tracy's clients loved that little boy—my clients, not so much. I think if I had not

chosen to leave that salon during that time, I would have lost a bunch of them. Good bye, bellowing boy!

LESSON LEARNED
Do what is best for you!

TRUSTING YOUR EMPLOYEE'S

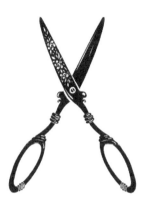

Rose was not a trusting boss. She stored all the perms in a locked closet. She would take out three at a time and place them in the dispensary. If you needed one or two, or more, for your day, you had to ask her or the manager for them. When Tracy was on maternity leave, Bonnie was the acting manager. She came back to work after being arrested and told us all it had to do with parking tickets, which I knew was a crock of shit.

Bonnie even had the extra key now. No matter what happened, Bonnie was a favorite of Rose's. But to be completely honest, Rose never trusted *any* employees.

One day, when I was walking across the parking lot to get change at the bank, *I caught her!* She had parked her van across from the bank's parking lot, and I could see her clearly. She was watching the shop with binoculars. No kidding! Now that is some serious espionage!

I sighed and thought to myself... *I know I have not worked for her that long, but I'm out of here as soon as I can get another job!* Between Bonnie and her drama and Rose on stake out, this was too much for me.

Bonnie soon got in lots more trouble with the law and decided to make changes. She quit Action Salon and moved out of state, but I also heard the college football tight end was moving his sweet ass to play pro ball. I think this had something to do with her move, too.

A few days after Bonnie packed up her stuff and left, the shop was broken into. All the money Rose stored in the salon was gone. All Rose's things had been ransacked—chemicals, perms, color, even shears of Rose's were gone. (Odd, because none of my things were missing, nor Mary's or Jo's. But Tracy's nice expensive shears, clippers, blow dryer and curling iron's were all gone.)

It was so obvious that it was Bonnie, but Rose would never admit her sweet Bonnie would do this. I'm thankful she did not touch my stuff, but looking back—who would want beauty school shears and the beauty school rollers with #56 on them?

One evening when closing the till, I was off by a dollar and a few cents. I was too tired to figure it out; it was almost ten o'clock and I needed to be back in by nine in the morning. I decided to let it slide until morning and to go ahead and make the deposit in the drop box at the bank.

The next day, I arrived to see Rose is already working on the difference from the closing from the night before. She was not happy. I had gotten there early to figure this out, and I was not sure why she was so upset over this small amount.

Maybe it was the last straw. Maybe it was that she and I had never seen eye-to-eye. I was not going to kiss her big ass over this. I will never know what drove her distrust of me and other employees, but after that, every day I looked for an opportunity to get my big ass out of there.

LESSON LEARNED
Some bosses are better than others!

Kimberly McBee

THANKFUL TO BE MOVING ON

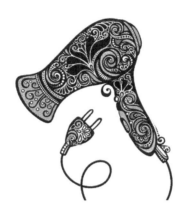

When working in a salon, I could be an employee, I could lease and be an independent operator, or own. I figured since I was always fully booked, it gave me the confidence and the money I needed for the next step—it was time to rent a station and become an independent operator. Without delay, I got my independent license. I was already licensed by the state, so it wasn't hard to get; I just had to apply. I did have to carry insurance, but it felt like no biggie to become my own boss. I was excited.

    I had this on my mind when I was sitting at the bar in the local Marie Callender's restaurant, a favorite hangout for Mark and me. They had free appetizers as long as you were drinking, and the best long island ice teas. They served the long islands in what we called "a fishbowl," but you might call them a frosted glass schooner. They also served fresh veggies and sometimes they had a yummy taco bar.

I ate tons and tons of broccoli and ranch at that time. My iron count was better then—and so was my waistline.

Long Island's are mostly alcohol and not much in calories. But, I figured these drinks were helping me build up my tolerance for alcohol! *Yes, I'm Kim and I like to drink, but no Mom, I'm not an alcoholic.* (My mother was worried.)

As I sat there sipping my drink, I was checking the want ads in the local paper while Mark and some friends were talking. We were bellying up to the bar, and I saw an ad for a hair station for rent at a tanning salon. It was only a few miles from the shop where I currently worked.

I looked at the date of the paper. It was old. *Damn it!* I thought to myself… *I'm sure it's already taken.* I got up and called anyway, and Shannon the owner was not there, but I was told to just come in the next day and drop off a resumé.

Here I go again—the next morning I dressed to my best ability and walked into the Tanning Salon with my resume and a smile. I wonder which is more important?

The manager at the front desk looked like she should be in a Van Halen music video with her long, blonde, curly hair. She was beautiful.

"Hi," she said with a smile. I looked around, intrigued by this place, which I had never been in before. It seemed hip and new—and totally different from anywhere I had ever worked. It reminded me of some type of place you would see in California. There were colorful, trendy clothes and sexy bikinis, tanning oils, and mini glasses to protect your eyes from the tanning bed rays.

The front desk was placed in the center bow of the tanning salon, with its glass block bottom. I walked to the back and there were six tanning bed stalls, three on each side. Painted in blue and greens, it was very tropical. *It felt happy!*

The bathroom was in the back left corner of the store. To the right, was an office for the manager or owner. The manager showed me the hair station, a cube-like area right between the bathroom and office. The station was open with no door. To the left, closest to the bathroom, glass blocks were stacked six feet tall. This was a really pretty area; I watched the light glimmer into the station.

I walked on into the station with its' blue lament top and wet bar. The shampoo bowl was under the table top. The hinged table lifted up, and the stylist simply had to swivel the chair, and lean the client back for a shampoo, then have them sit back up. Behind that, there were cabinets, colored in the same pretty blue. Locked cabinets, so I would be able to safely store my tools, color, perms etc.

I loved it—the whole set up—and I lightheartedly asked the manager, "When can I start?" I was so confident I was a good fit for this job, I forgot I was just dropping off the resume!

About that time, Shannon, the owner, walked in. She was a five-feet-six—a young brunette. She was sweet and pretty, with a runner's body. We greeted, and would have shaken hands, but her hands were full.

"I'll put these things in the office and be right out," she told me. She was older than me, but not that much older. At this time, I was twenty-four, and had been married for two years. Shannon was around twenty-nine.

She smiled and asked, "Can you start today?" We laughed and talked of many things for about an hour. I told her that I need to give two weeks notice.

She explained there was a woman booked this evening that she could use my help with if I was able to do it. She had hired a young woman who had just finished Beauty College—and at the last minute she had gotten scared and decided not to take the job. But the problem was—Shannon had already booked Ms. Just Finished Beauty College a perm.

After thinking about it for a minute, I said, "I can do it."

She was so pleased that she let out an excited little, yip! "Oh, thank you, I hate calling people and disappointing them."

I looked over the appointment book with Shannon, and planned to come back in a few hours to do my first guest in the new station. I was so excited and could not wait. I thought… *this is perfect!*

This meant more money for me, plus a nice manager and great atmosphere. I was so excited to lease a station and be my own boss. The rent was $350 a month—and it was up to me—I could work as much or as little as I liked. I had received my independent license from the state, so I was prepared for this moment.

That evening, I came in carrying everything I needed to work on one client for a perm. (She arrived early, and was getting a manicure from one of the manicurists. Acrylic nails were becoming very popular in the early nineties.)

The Tanning Salon had more than one nail technician—and she was much better than any of my attempts at nails. I felt this client had money—she just reeked of it. She stood out to me, because I was used to the middle class clients where I had worked before.

I felt like I was a country girl who had just fallen off the hay truck, but I could not stop staring at her fingers dripping with diamonds. She was sweet as honey, but seemed unhappy. Her name was Melanie, and I talked and consulted with her.

She talked about her husband who had been a pilot. He had been working hard flying here and there for a commercial airline. He made great money, super career, and she did not have to work. She loved her life.

But then she shared with me how, recently, her world had come crashing down. Her wonderful husband was diagnosed with early-stage cancer. She needed a hairstyle that was low maintenance.

"I will not be able to come in as I usually have, and in fact, this is my last manicure for a while."

I examined Melanie and liked that she had such beautiful, thick, brownish hair. For lower maintenance, I thought it might be better not to perm her hair. And perms were not as much in style any longer. A shorter cut would make her look younger, and I could show her an easy way to style it with a little spray gel. She liked the idea of the no hassle style, but was not sure about not perming since she had been doing it for years.

I worked on Melanie's cut for an hour. She looked younger and I could tell that a weight had been lifted, even if it was just for an hour or so. I'm glad some people feel relief from their stressful situations during their time in the chair.

Melanie walked out of my new place of business and commented to Shannon, "You've got a winner."

I was so proud. *Ya Rose—Shannon got a winner when she hired me!*

When I told Rose I was moving on to be my own boss by leasing a station, she said something that I'll never ever forget. "YOU WILL JUST GET AUDITED."

I thought to myself... *When I have employees, I will never try to crush their dreams.*

So, this winner moved on, without hesitation.

LESSON LEARNED

Sometimes life throws curve balls, so swing for the fences! Taking a different road, sets you on a different path!

LEAVE THE OLD CHAIR START NEW

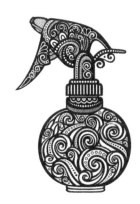

Two weeks notice and I would be out of Rose's salon. I reluctantly finished my time. Rose treated me as if I had the plague. I would rather have stopped altogether and moved straight into my new job and left this one behind me.

"I can do this!" I told myself. And in no time I began at the Tanning Salon. I loved it from day one; the women who worked there were my kind of people. Shannon was fun and full of life. I was making more money than I ever had, and I had clients coming out my wazoo! Frankly, this side of the freeway had more money and clients were hungry for skilled stylists with new techniques and insight.

I loved my job, and it kept me busy with people from all walks of life. One day, I was working on a new elderly client at the new salon and station. She told me all about herself, with no regard about time.

I couldn't get a word in edgewise to find out what she would like for her service. Just then Shannon walked through the salon and into her office with an attractive black fellow on her heel. "Oh, what is that all about?" the women in my chair asked.

I had to take another look to find out what she was talking about. "What do you mean ma'am?" She looked disgusted. "Why is that white woman going in that room with that black man?"

Well, I looked at her, a confused look on my face, "That is Shannon and she is the owner of this establishment and that is her office. I think that is a salesman, but I'm not sure. Is there a problem?"

The woman was so offended that she decided to leave. I had never experienced racism like this. I had no idea what she was really thinking; I couldn't relate, but it was as if he was raping this poor white woman in that back room. Thankfully, this racist woman left, with the door hitting her in the ass.

Shannon came out and I said "I do not want her back," and fortunately I never saw that ignorant woman again.

By the way, Shannon bought lights for the shop and several other products from this attractive and professional salesman over the years. He was a great guy; I became friends with him and got to know his wife, and did her hair for years.

Shh! She was a white, blonde-haired, blue-eyed beauty...

LESSON LEARNED
Ignorance in people is sad!

BEBOPPING BAMBI

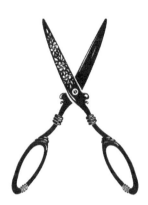

A young woman walked in for an appointment to have her hair bleached and styled, with no haircut. She was very voluptuous, her hair almost white from bleaching. Her roots were nearly black, so she asked me to put bleach on her roots, to even out her sexy locks.

I asked her name. The girls at the front had written it on my schedule, but their handwriting was not the best, so I didn't think I was reading it right.

She replied, "No worries, it's Bambi!"

I responded, "Bambi?"

"Ya, like the Disney character."

I finished big-boobed Bambi's hair, and she asked the cost. I totaled all the services and gave her a bill for eighty dollars.

She dug into her bright blue purse, and pulled out a handful of single dollar bills. They were crumpled. She began to straighten them while she counted, one at a time. She actually had eighty singles, plus twenty others, she handed me one hundred of the "George" greenbacks.

Just then, I saw Bambi for who she really was, or at least I realized what she did for a living. I had taken off my gloves I wore for applying hair color and wished I had not. I didn't want to touch this hard-earned cash. I asked her to set it down on the counter and acted like I was cleaning up, even though the clean up had already been done.

Bambi thanked me and bebopped down the hall to the outside door with her bouncing bombshell blonde curls. I slipped on some new form-fitting latex gloves and picked up the dollars and walked to the front desk where the owner of the salon, Shannon was sitting. "Could you possibly use some ones?" I asked.

She said "Sure." Someone paid with a hundred dollar bill, you want that?" she asked.

"That would be great!" I said. I did not tell Shannon that the dollar exchange came from a stripper. Shannon took them, glad to have the change—as she tucked them neatly in the register.

YUCK!

LESSON LEARNED
Keep your gloves on 'cause you never know where the greenbacks have been.

MARY JANE

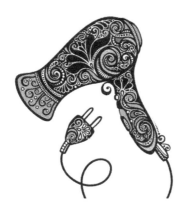

I was enjoying working full time at my leased station behind the sparkling glass blocks. The salon had an island feel.

A new client, Mary Jane walked in. She was an elementary teacher. She wanted to make an appointment to have a consultation. I happened to have ten minutes, so we were able to talk right then in front of the mirror.

I looked at her blonde mullet. It was a Rod Stewart look-alike hairstyle; kind of spiked on top. She was pretty upset. A male sylist at another salon had taken his aggressions out on her poor little head.

We laughed a little as we talked, even though I knew she was a little teary-eyed. One bad cut is like wearing an ugly outfit every day. I told her as gently as I could that we needed to cut the back off. She could not have the varied lengths. The goal was to grow out some of the top, with it cut into a cute bob. This would be the most becoming with her fine limp hair. Too many layers can make hair collapse.

She was willing, so we made an appointment for the next day. She wanted it immediately, and I couldn't blame her, but the client who was on my book was already waiting.

The next day rolled around and it was time for Mary Jane's appointment. She came in with a friend who wanted a consultation. So I cut Mary Jane's hair first.

Her friend, Kathy, was a kick. She had finer hair than M.J. and she still wanted to leave the length. I suggested color. It swells the hair shaft and makes strands feel fat. She made an appointment. Mary Jane paid; I thanked her for bringing in a friend.

To this day, Mary Jane is one of my most valuable clients (MVC). *Thank you, Mary Jane!*

For years, she has sent in friends to me. I thank her for such loyalty and great referrals. I hope she knows how much she helped me when I was just starting in my new chair adventure.

LESSON LEARNED
Some clients are worth their weight in gold!

PEEPING TOM

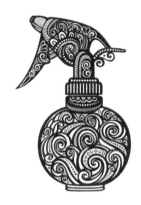

At the Tanning Salon, I remember working to the beat of six different radio stations all at once; back then we didn't have headphones. The nail fumes were pretty strong, but for the most the part perm fumes were gone!

It was a beautiful place, full of color—even the shades on the patrons with their golden tans looked good. Though to be honest, I hated to see new people start tanning. They would go in not understanding how easily they could get burnt, *and burnt bad*—not knowing what that could mean for their skin.

The owner hired young beauties to work at the front desk. I think long hair and big breasts were a requirement. Some were beautiful and smart, but most did not have a lot upstairs. All boobs and no brains. Answering phones, taking appointments, cleaning tanning beds and keeping the place neat and clean was their job.

There were a few different women working at the front desk. I liked the single ones best, because they did not hang all over their boyfriends up front or talk endlessly on the phone with their boy toys.

One day while I was working in the back, Shannon sent in her guy friend to watch the front. (She let him use the tanning beds for free.) The shop was not too busy, and the gal for the next shift was sick. It did not take long to figure out that he was in love with Shannon and she knew it, and she used this to her advantage.

He was a quite a pro whenever he worked the front reception desk. He flirted with any girl that came in young, old, pretty, or not so pretty. I think he made plenty of sales on swimwear, lotions and potions.

However, something unusual happened that particular evening. One of the university cheerleaders came in for a tan. She was a Bella (a beauty). Long blonde hair with natural curl and bronze skin—and big, I mean huge, blue eyes. I saw her step into the tanning station and shut the door.

But the unusual thing was the silence... except for her radio and the noise I was making as I cleaned up for my next client. I was tired... *She will be my last* I kept telling myself and my aching feet.

About that time, my client walked in the front door and I heard her shriek. "WHAT ARE YOU DOING UP THERE?"

You guessed it, Shannon's front desk, fill-in friend, aka "Peeping Tom" was watching this young unknowing cheerleader as she lay there soaking up the tanning rays with her little spacey-looking tanning eye wear.

Tanning in the nude is normal. Tanning while some guy is hanging over the edge of the tanning wall is not. My client caught him red-handed.

That was an interesting appointment for my client. (Thank God I knew her!) She has never forgotten that appointment day; me either.

P.S. We never let the cheerleader know about Peeping Tom.

He quickly jumped down and pretended nothing had happened; I took my client back to do her hair trying not to make a bigger deal of it, since it was bad enough.

He was never able to work in the Tanning Salon again. He should never be able to come in and work at all, but that was just my opinion. I didn't own the place.

LESSON LEARNED
Don't ever hire perverts.

Kimberly McBee

ELDERS

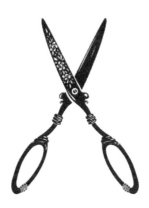

I was taught to respect my elders—and I learned to enjoy the older generation at work and play.

A lot of the "older" (WW II) generation had their hair done once a week back in the day. I was taught how to back-comb and do traditional roller placement. I had a Friday morning full of these sweet ladies. Bread and butter, as you will. You could always rely on them. They never bounced checks. They never did a "no show" unless they had an emergency. Usually a sudden death of a friend or pet is the reason they would miss a hair appointment. Reliable!

But I learned that once you do their hair each week, you have to start entertaining them. So... I shared things about my life with them. They loved hearing that I wanted to start a family. I told them: Mark and I are going to buy a new home. I talked about our vacations, my relationship with family members, and the parties Mark and I liked to throw. They enjoyed the hour in my chair—time away from their housework. They relaxed while sitting under the warm dryer—while they read their smut. That's their word, not mine. *PEOPLE Magazine,* SMUT!

Some elders are all business and just want their hair done, but over time some become family. I'm always sad when one leaves this earth, but they can't live forever. I know that one day my time is coming too. I'll probably be working behind the chair and just drop!

LESSON LEARNED
There has to be a place where you look great all the time and your feet don't ache!

SUDDEN "SHARESIES"

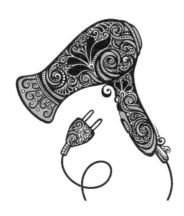

I first met Jewels when she walked into the salon one day—and she threw me for a loop. Dressed very professionally, she was wearing a skirt and collared blouse, and her heels echoed on the floor as she confidently walked across the room. Her hair was perfect and her nails were colorfully manicured. She appeared older than me. (Me? I was dressed in shorts and sandals, since I'm pretty laid back when I work.)

She introduced herself, and without a pause said, "We needed to figure out our schedules."

I had absolutely no clue what she was talking about. "What schedules? And who are you again?" I asked.

"I'm Jewels. My sister-in-law does nails here and I'm going to be sharing the hair station with you."

I had worked here for six months and rented the station. I had not asked for a workmate. I hadn't had good luck with women roommates, so sharing a hair station was not high on my list. I told her I didn't know what she was talking about.

She went on to tell me that she and Shannon had talked about this. Apparently Jewels was leaving a job at J.C. Penny's salon to come here and share my station. As I listened to her tale, I tried to be cool, but inside I was outraged.

I stomped off to find Shannon, but was unable to talk to her. She was in the back room with one of the new massage therapists. She had built onto the Tanning Salon, and there were now four nail stations and a back room for facials and massages.

I was furious that Shannon would do this without even telling me. I walked back over to where Jewels was standing, and she had her schedule book in hand. I took a deep breath. I listened to her tell me she would be using the nail station in front of the salon area and also do hair part time *in my station.*

I asked, "How many hours will you need?"

She casually said, "I'm pretty flexible. I can work anytime you are not there.

My schedule was Tuesday through Saturday. She was already making faces. "What?" I asked, already getting tired of the look on her face.

She pushed her point. "I work Saturday's too."

"Oh," was all I could think to say for a second. My thoughts were scrambling every which way. "Maybe we could work every other Saturday, I have been working Saturdays for years. I would like a Saturday off once in a while."

Suddenly, I see Shannon heading our way towards her office after her massage. She saw Jewels talking with me, and turned a 180, and walked in the opposite direction.

I ignored her, because by this point I knew she had done this. It was not right. If she would have just told me, we could have worked it out.

But as I got to know Jewels, even with her perfect look and assertiveness seemed pretty cool.

Without a word from Shannon, Jewels and I worked out our work schedules. We decided to work every other Saturday and she would work Monday as much as she liked. The rest of the week we shared. I had Friday all to myself, but Tuesday, Wednesday, and Thursday I either worked morning, and she worked the night shift, or she worked the morning and I worked the night shift. This ended up being a team made in heaven.

Thanks, Shannon! We made it work, and work well.

Jewels became pregnant after about two years of us sharing the station. I helped her out by taking some of her loyal clientele. She helped me out one day when I went skiing and did not make it down the hill with all my gear intact. I created a garage sale on the snow slopes. My left knee will never be the same. I tore my ACL—and it ended up being the nasty surgery that changed my life. Volleyball was definitely not going to be in my life as much, and skiing the slopes was now a bigger challenge. But… I could still stand and work behind the chair!

LESSON LEARNED
Don't get too cocky on the ski slopes!

Kimberly McBee

MICE

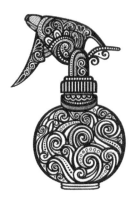

The last year in our little shack, we started having mice in our house. The last straw was what happened in the garage one day. I opened the washer and saw what I thought was a sock on the side of the washer drum, But no, it was a friggin mouse! I picked it up still thinking it was a wet sock. It was a mouse, a stinking mouse!

I looked at it and screamed! I think it looked back at me and screamed as well. I dropped the poor squiggling little gray mouse and ran into the house.

In the paper, I found an ad "Free to good home: three cats." I called about the cats and went to see them. I drove fifteen minutes out to see the freebies, knowing a cat could help us with our mice problem.

We lived in front of a cherry orchard and the momma mice wanted to come in and have their babies in our little garage. Free cats could solve the mice problem.

I arrived at the address. The driveway had an old car that looked like it had been there for a very long time. I could see a barking dog that looked like he could eat me alive. I thought, "CUJO!"

I parked as close to the house as possible, but there were a few cars already ahead of me. I knocked and a man opened the door. I told him I had come to see the cats.

"Come on in, " he said.

"Yeah, they're in here." We walked into the main family room and I saw the ugliest kitty-cat that I had ever seen. There was a family trying to decide if they wanted this poor excuse for a kitten.

Suddenly down the stairs came a fluffy Himalayan blue-eyed feline. I asked the owner if she was one of the cats they were getting rid of.

"Yeah, " he said, being exasperated at the family that could not make up their mind.

I nearly yelled "I'll take her!" The Himalayan must not have come down the stairs before now, because the family saw her and said, "AAH!"

I quickly took my beauty to the car and put her in a pet carrier. Obviously, she had not been in a car or a pet carrier before. She howled all the way to her new home.

She was a wonderful find. I named her Miss Kitty. She made all the mice *magically* disappear in no time.

LESSON LEARNED
Hang on to memories, not mice!

NEW HOUSE

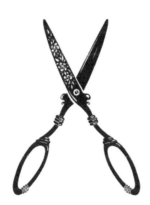

We wanted to sell the little shack we had lived in for seven years, to move closer to the city of Eugene where we both worked. Bandit, our first born (the dog) had been rented out to "THE SLUT" for stud service.

We began to think moving him into town was a bad idea. We had not been able to keep him home. He ran away a lot—he was quite the man about town. One day, I scoured the country neighborhood trying to find him. A woman walked out of her trailer house and I asked her, "Have you seen a beagle running around here?"

She quickly replied. "Oh, him!" "He was the father of our last batch of puppies."

I looked at her little pooch, a long-haired miniature poodle, and thought... *Yikes, those must have been ugly puppies!*

So... we decided it was best to find Bandit a good home in the country. His new home was on one hundred acres and he had three females to hump. What else could he ask for? I was not sad for him, due to the fact he was inheriting a harem. We had another beagle, a female, that we had gotten a few years before, and had a few litters of pups.

One year, we sold them at Christmas time. It was fun finding them good homes, and watching young people come pick out their new baby beagle. There was a young blind woman who picked out one. It was her Christmas present from her boyfriend. I had a young boy come for his very first puppy. Special! We also made a little Christmas money to spend on each other when we sold the puppies for fifty bucks each.

Millie was the name of our female beagle. She was black and white and not full bred. We loved her. She was a slob and not very lady like at all. She ate all her food and Bandits too, if we did not feed them separately. I decided to have her fixed so she was unable to have any more litters. She got an infection, and unfortunately she did not survive. Rest in peace, aka Pig Dog; we loved you.

On we went… we painted our little shack and cleaned the carpets and put up a "For Sale" sign in the yard.

In three days we had five buyers—one offer and four back up offers. The first one fell through. The second one backed out. The third one couldn't qualify. The fourth one went through, and we got what we asked for it. Full price!

I was excited, because we had made an offer on a brand new home. Since the shack sold in three days, our dream to have a new home was coming true. I wanted to do cartwheels in the front room.

We went from 720 square feet to 1640 square feet—white carpets, beige walls, and lots of windows. The neighborhood we moved to had lots of young families. We did not have children yet, but it was not from a lack of trying. Mark and I wanted children, but had not yet been blessed.

We moved in with hardly any furniture to fill the home. We had some old, hand-me-downs. We were in a brand spanking-new home, and using these old items made it look shabby chic. That is what I told myself, because I could not afford anything else.

LESSON LEARNED
Appreciate what you have.

Kimberly McBee

BABIES

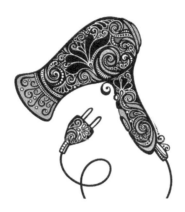

I wanted to start a family. Young women came in all the time, but when I wanted to have a baby, they seemed to be the only ones to get pregnant. We began to think, "BABIES ARE NOT IN THE CARDS FOR US!"

Mark and I looked at all the reasons why—or rather, why not! I took eveyone's advice. My grandmother had me take Vitamin E. "Stand on your head after sex." She told me more than once. I decided to see a doctor, and I told Mark to switch from briefs to boxers.

The doctor's office did not offer me much information or help. The specialist just wanted to sell me on very expensive fertility treatments. He reminded me of a car salesman. He was determined to sell me on this in-vitro process. This meant I would have to get a regimen of shots, and also take my temp every time, to see the right time for me and Mark to make whoopee. That took all the fun out of it.

I wanted answers. I didn't know why this was happening. We had been married for six years and had not used birth control during all those years, so why, oh why was this infertility happening to us?

The doctor just told us my body did not do what needed to happen to produce a baby. So I started with Clomid, an infertility drug. This pill makes a woman's body ovulate. I was a crazy person on this medication. Mark could not stand to be in the same room with me, let alone make a baby with me. I decided right there and then, we were not meant to have children. We stopped all pills. We both put it in our minds that we were not going to be a family of three or four, but a family of two.

Our new home was beautiful. Since no babies were in our future, maybe it was time to move on and create my own salon.

LESSON LEARNED
Once again... life has a way of reminding us to appreciate what we have!

CHILDREN HAVING CHILDREN

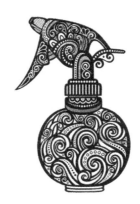

Chrissy, a new client, came in to get a haircut. I noticed right away she was pregnant. I asked her if it was a boy or girl. "It's a boy; I'm not too excited," she said while holding up her ankles that looked like they could explode.

"You look like you are retaining some water," I said.

"You think?" Chrissy was not yet twenty. I was guessing that this was not a planned pregnancy.

I talked with Chrissy and we figured out she just wanted a trim and a braid to get the hair off her sticky neck. Chrissy had wonderful skin, no wrinkles, and no scars; perfect. It was the golden tan color many women want, and she had pretty blue eyes with black eyelashes that I would give my left boob for.

"I don't want a baby?" Chrissy told me.

I wanted to cry out "Well I DO!" I had been married for six and one-half years, and still, no luck. Here, this young, beautiful woman was pregnant with a child that she was not wanting or prepared for. I wasn't judging, because believe me, I'm not perfect; I admit I felt jealous. I wanted a baby so badly, and as she sat in my chair pregnant, it was a harsh reminder that felt like a slap in the face. I told her I had been trying forever, and she told me that if she decided to give this baby up she would let me know.

My heart skipped a beat, not because of the chance that I could adopt her baby, but how she was so disingenuous towards this new unborn human being that was a part of her. I finished her cut and braid and she paid. She told me we would keep in touch. I gave her my business card.

A year later, here came Chrissy again, but this time I was cutting little Jason's hair. We sat him in a booster seat and all I could think of was this baby could have been mine. Obviously Chrissy did not give up her baby boy for adoption. She decided to keep the bright little man. He was born bald, and it took about a year before he needed a trim on his pretty little head. (The thing is, those bald babies seem to be the people with the most hair as adults.)

I kept in contact with Chrissy, cutting her hair for years, and watched her have more than one child while I still could not conceive a child. It was time to think of other things to occupy my time.

LESSON LEARNED
Babies are special, whether they are yours or belong to someone else.

HONEYCOMB

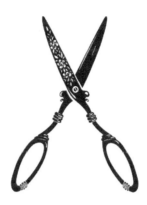

We now lived in our big new house—and we were really enjoying it. We loved mowing the lawn, or at least Mark loved mowing the lawn. He did it about every two or three days. He was proud of this perfectly manicured grass. I planted jasmine and a few lilac bushes. This home fulfilled our dream.

My next dream was to own my own salon. I was looking at different areas, and different properties to put in a brand new salon. I wanted it to be close to our house.

I got a call one afternoon from the realtor that had helped us sell our little shack. She also had helped us get into our new home. I laughed, thinking... *she had not made enough money from us that year,* so she told me... "I found a salon for you!" She was so excited, she was hard to understand, but I was listening intently.

I asked, "What have you found?

She had found a salon that was for sale two

miles from our new home. She told me "You can buy the land and the salon.

I thought to myself… *right, like we can afford that!*

I guess it's all about timing, because my grandmother had passed away some time before this and had left each one of us (her grandchildren) a little something. That is the money I had to put into a salon of my own.

I told the real-estate agent that I would love to take a look. We made an appointment with the agent that was handling the salon for the owners. We went to see it a few evenings later—and it really was only two miles from our new house. It was a small 1930s home. It was white on the outside with blue trim. It had a front porch with a wheelchair ramp, and had been converted into a full salon. No living quarters.

It had a driveway wide enough for two cars, and then it opened in the back with a gravel lot, with enough room for up to ten vehicles.

As I went up two steps onto a small porch, I liked the windowed door. As we walked in a buzzer went off, not too loud, but enough so you knew someone walked in.

The shop was PINK. I mean Pepto-Bismol PINK! The walls and shampoo bowls were also pink; the floor was off white with pink flowers.

The back door opened into a very short corridor. To the left was the kitchen (break room/dispensary.) To the right were the two shampoo bowls, pink no less!

What used to be the front room of the house had

the front desk and two hair stations. In the middle of the shop was a tiny hall that led back to two more stations. As I walked to the right, there was a hallway with a hot water heater closet. To the right of this was the one stool bathroom, and to the left was another room which the current owner used for five hood dryers—and it was also used for a book exchange.

My first impression was that it was dark in the house, but then I was looking at it when it was dark outside. I thought it was cute, but I didn't like the wicker furniture in the waiting room. I definitely didn't dig all the pink. The pink shampoo bowls were kinda' cool though.

In one of the front stations, there was a huge stain on the floor. I wasn't sure if it was hair color or water damage. There were a lot of windows, but with it being nighttime, I couldn't tell if the daylight would make the house light and bright.

The glass front door gave me a great view of the two beautiful ornamental cherry trees in front; they had fluffy soft pink springtime blossoms. These things might sell me on the salon: Great parking. Great visibility. Very convenient to where we lived.

We talked to the agent handling the sale, and then two more people walked in, a man and a woman in their fifties. They spotted me, and almost gave me the impression that they felt this was a waste of their time. I was twenty-nine and so was Mark. This would be a huge investment, but we felt prepared to take it on.

We sat down to discuss the cost, and the woman who owned it shared what she was thinking. She wanted to stay on as an employee. I was not too sure this was a great idea. I figured we could always do it on a trial basis and see how it worked out. They could see I was serious.

We did it! We sold our first home, bought a brand new home, and bought our first business, all in the same year.

The shop was named Honeycomb Hair Salon. I did not like the name, but there were clients already coming in the door, so I left the name—but probably not for long. With me bringing in my former clients and all the current clients still walking in the door, how could I go wrong? Turn key!

LESSON LEARNED
Always know what you are walking into!

BIG BAD BOSS – ME!

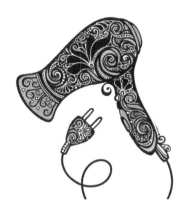

First day on the job, I dressed the part and showed up on time. I walked in to get the key from the past owner. The three women who worked there also came in to meet me. There were four stations and four employees, besides the previous owner.

The stylist in the front station had black hair and one chipped front tooth. Why in this day and age would you not fix a chipped tooth when you work in the beauty industry?

Her face turned beet red when the women were all told that Casey had sold the shop. I was not liked at all on that first day!

The girl in the back room station was pregnant and I could see she would be off work having that bundle of joy soon; maybe tomorrow. Her voice was so loud that I could not hear myself think. The third woman was older than the rest, and she seemed kind and positive, when the other two were not. I found out this was the first they had heard of the shop being for sale, let alone sold. I guess their surprise was taken out on me. Hey, I was innocent. All I had done was buy the business and property. *If you are not nice you do not need to stay,* I thought.

But I did not have to fire anyone; the chipped tooth quit two days after I took ownership of the shop. Good riddance. The pregnant woman went on maternity leave a week later, and then after the baby was born, she went on to drive a school bus. I was glad. A week of her loud voice in that little salon was way too much for this girl.

Two weeks into working the new salon I planned to do a grand opening. Jewels called me from the Tanning Salon; she was tired of all the receptionists not doing their job, and the station rent going up. She decided to move to my salon; she took over the station next to me. She worked as an independent operator, leasing the station from me.

Casey, the previous owner, stayed on part time, and the kind older woman also stayed with us. All stations were full. The remodel changes were very slow in coming. I tried not to scare off our clients that already walking in the door.

I did get rid of the artificial flowers in the bathroom after one of my first clients went to the restroom and asked me, "Who died?" The first change was made then and there. We detailed the yard and made it look neat and pretty.

This salon had charged eleven dollars for a haircut, but at that time at the Tanning Salon I was charging twenty-two dollars and was not about to go down on my prices, so I just did it—I changed the prices and no one seemed to blink an eye.

They had been charged for every little thing, so the customers appreciated not being "nickeled and dimed." My costs were straightforward and understood.

I realized Casey had watered down the back bar shampoo. She bought perms that were beauty college quality—not the best—and anyone could identify them from the putrid smell as soon as they walked into the salon.

LESSON LEARNED
Treat individuals as you want to be treated and avoid using cheap products—cheap is cheap!

Kimberly McBee

ROAD TRIP

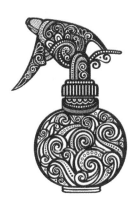

After the grand opening, my doors were officially open; we all worked hard. Since Jewels was now working with us, I made her the manager. She was someone I trusted, and to this day I do not know if she knows how I feel about her—a Soul Sister, I would say.

I had a client who had lived in Vegas, and had moved to Oregon to be close to her grandchildren. I did her hair once a week—styling, cutting, and coloring when needed.

After doing her hair for less than a year, she told me she was moving back to Vegas. "I don't see my kids or my grandkids any more, whether I live here or in Vegas," she said. So she told me and all the girls at the salon to look her up if we came to Vegas!

Two weeks passed, and on the one year anniversary of the salon I asked Jewels if she wanted to take a road trip to Vegas over a long weekend. She told me she was in. No one else wanted to join us, so the shop stayed open while we were gone. My younger sister wanted to go, since she was single and fancy free.

The three of us packed and ended up driving my Honda Accord. We decided to drive in shifts and try to drive all night. As we drove over the mountain to the east it was dark. We were driving in fog that you could cut with a knife. I was at the wheel and saw two headlights coming toward us, but I thought it was my eyes playing tricks on me.

He is coming straight for us. Oh no, he was in my lane and this semi-truck was either asleep or playing chicken with us! I swerved to the right as his lights hit my front bumper. We were wide awake then—and our adrenaline hit at an all time high... but safe... *WHEW!*

We drove and drove, *and drove,* to make it to Reno, Nevada. There were tiny little creatures running across the road as I was driving, and I thought they had a death wish! I hit none, but I don't know why not. Maybe I was just tired and they were a figment of my imagination.

My parents were visiting Reno, so we decided to stop and rest. We arrived at their hotel room as they got back from late-night gambling. We told them how tired we were, so even though it was early morning, they said they would go out again and let us rest in their room for a few hours. All three of us climbed into the same huge bed and slept for a couple of hours.

We woke and ate breakfast with my mother and

father—and piled into my Honda and took off again. I'm sure my parents thought... *finally, some sleep!* "ZZZ's...!"

On we went—again we drove and drove. We saw a blinking beer sign in a window. Jewels needed to call her new man, and I thought I better call Mark, too. We stopped at what we thought was a little store. They had a convenient pay phone on the outside. (There weren't cell phones back then; at least we didn't have them.)

We walked up to the front door to grab a coke or a snack from the store. All three of us entered the front door. There was a second door to enter into the inside *of the store.* Jewels, Keri and I read the sign posted on the wall: **Condoms Must Be Worn, State Law. Required.** It hit us all at the same time. Keri hurtled over the top of me to get out of there and back to the car.

You guessed it! Unknown to us, we were entering a brothel. "The Cotton Tail Ranch..." Only then did we see the huge sign. I started the car... so much for making a phone call...

We learned that you could have one of the girls come out to the car or have them get ready in a room... *Maybe an order to go? Who knows!*

We saw a man drive in with his horse trailer hitched to the back of his pick-up truck. There were two or three kids sitting in his truck. He ran inside carrying something.

I don't know... my best guess was he was taking his working wife lunch! Second guess: A quickie while the kids waited?

Maybe we should have gotten an application?

LESSON LEARNED
Read signs for content.

INSPECTOR

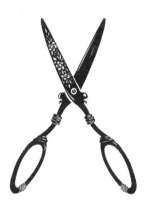

A salon requires a state license, and the state inspector can come at any time to inspect it—without notice.

I had owned the salon for four years, and had always seemed to dodge being there when the inspector came in. Not on purpose. It was either my day off or I was out running errands.

My manager just happened to be the one working when he had come in, up until now. But on this particular day of his visit the shop was packed. I had a client in my chair and one waiting. My manager had a patron in her chair and one waiting, and there was a wedding party in the back getting a consult.

Kids were running around waiting for their mommies to get their hair styled. The massage therapist was doing a massage in the back room. It was just one of the crazy days.

The front door opened, and a man walked in

with his clipboard. I saw him and thought, *WHY NOW?*

I looked over at Jewels, my manager, and said, "Hey, are you good?" She gave me a thumbs up. I was basically asking if she had a clean station and if her licensing was all up to date.

I caught the attention of the girls in the back of the salon and told them an inspector was here. They looked like they had just seen a ghost. They were now in action. They began cleaning up combs on counters, and brushes they had been working with, and sweeping up hair and making everything tidy. Not that our shop was dirty. In fact, Tabitha from "Tabitha's Take Over," the T.V. show, would think it was clean. But with our day being crazy busy, an inspector could even write us up for not being as organized as we should be.

I decided to stall. I asked him how could I help him. I said, "We are pretty busy, so I don't know if we can take a walk-in right now."

He said to me "I'm not here for a haircut." As he spoke, he looked like he was in pain.

I asked him, "Are you okay?"

He said, gritting his teeth, "Do you have a bathroom?" I showed him the door to the restroom and told him to take his time. He shut the door and I heard the sounds of relief.

The girls were running around and even the clients were helping with the clean up. I checked the sanitizers and they were great. By the time the door opened from the bathroom, the shop was spotless and ready for inspection. The man came out. All I smelled was the orange spray that was suppose to cover up stinkiness in the bathroom.

So, again, I greeted the inspector. He was already writing on an evaluation sheet. He signed it and handed it to me, "The shop looks great!"

He handed me the paper, embarrassed as hell, he quickly left. As the door closed, the laughter I heard from the women was infectious.

We never saw that inspector again.

LESSON LEARNED
When you've gotta' go—you've gotta' go!

Kimberly McBee

Lessons Learned Behind the Chair

PIXIE MAN

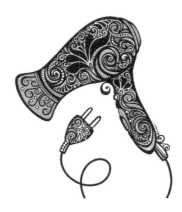

The first time Pixie Man called was the first year I owned the salon. He asked, "Do you know how to do a pixie cut?" I told him that I did and he asked, "Can you tell me how you would do this?"

So, not thinking anything about the question I answered him and described a pixie. "It's a short cut, no hair on the ears and pretty much short all over." He seemed satisfied and made appointments for his two daughters that he said were going sailing with him over the summer. They wanted an easy cut to hold up for the two months they would be away. The time came for their appointment and they didn't show up.

One year later, a man calls again. "Do you know how to cut a pixie cut?" He sounded fairly familiar, but I thought he was just a returning customer. Again, I explained the pixie cut and he made appointments for his two daughters.

Again, no show. One year later, I swear to the date, he called again. This time I remembered him, and confronted his no-shows and he hung up.

One year later Pixie Man called again—and the year after that and the year after that. Each employee was told about Pixie Man and it became almost a special time. If one of us got the call we would put him on hold and yell to the rest of the shop, "Pixie Man is calling!"

We would all gather around while he was put on speaker. The stories started. Some of the girls actually thought he did have two daughters that had pixie cuts and that they did go on this sailing adventure.

I just thought… *he's coo coo.*

The last time he called I asked him why he kept calling year after year and never showed up for the appointments? I was hoping to finally get an answer.

But, no. HE HUNG UP and was never heard from again!

LESSON LEARNED
Sometimes you just never know the full story!

TRAILER TRASH

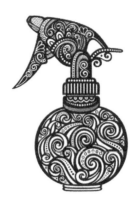

The back door opened, the bell went off, and a woman walked in. I looked up and saw a woman who had been in once before with her blind husband. They were neighbors of our manager. She never looked like she took much pride in what she was wearing or even combed her hair.

This day, she had her little daughter with her. She wanted to get her daughter's hair cut. My last patron, I sat her in a booster seat, even though I could have gone home instead. She was a tiny little thing. Her mom, not so much. She was tall and heavy set, with greasy, stringy hair. I even noticed an unpleasant odor.

I went ahead and draped the youngster and took one look at her greasy hair. I saw live lice crawling on her head, not just a few, she was infested. I told her mom, "I cannot cut her hair today."

We were the only ones left in the salon, so I

talked very frank with her about the lice. Otherwise, I would have taken her to the back room and spoken with her more discreetly. I told her she needed to be treated, explaining that I could cut her daughter's hair when she was lice free.

I looked a little closer and saw an open wound on the child's scalp. "What happened?" I asked.

The mother rolled her eyes, "She fell from her tree fort."

I looked at the little girl's face and thought, "I bet she has a concussion."

I told her that I felt she needed medical attention, and the mother was not happy that I was suggesting she take her daughter to the doctor. They left. (I would have loved to take this little one and give her a different life. It's sad: You have to have a license to drive, a license to do hair, but anyone can have children.)

I did not see Trailer Trash for a long time, until one day she came into the shop to get a perm for herself. A new employee that I had hired ended up giving her a spiral curl.

This new employee looked great and had lots of qualifications. However, the first day on the job she wore a short, short skirt so if she bent over you could tell she was female. No questions asked. I did not know how many tattoos she had but there were more than ten. She hid them well during the interview, not that I would have cared, but why would you hide who you are and then show up the first day, exposing more than just tattoos?

Oh well… back to the perm. My new employee did a fine job. One year later: The same trailer trash woman walks in and by now the employee that had permed her hair had moved out of the city and no longer worked for me. The woman looked like she had just crawled out of bed. I greeted her at the front desk. The shop once again was packed. My next guest was in the waiting area watching as I talked to this greasy haired, unkempt looking woman. (I never did see her little girl again.)

She said "I want to get a new perm. The girl that permed my hair said it would last a year and it's not even been a year yet."

I looked at her like she had to be kidding. "Let me look up your card" I said. I looked up her record card. There it was. A perm was given to her almost one year, to date, maybe shy by a week or so.

I looked at her hair and told her she still had some curl, but just needed a cut.

She asked if the cut was going to be free.

"No." Even though it had been nearly one year, I also told her that we guaranteed our perms for one month as long as a person uses our recommended shampoo and conditioner.

She stood in front of the reception desk blinking like she did not understand what I had just said. I repeated myself and then told her there was no one that can give a full year guarantee on a perm.

She said to me, "The girl who permed my hair did!" I explained that she still had curl, and just needed a shaping and that would pick up her curl. She was not happy with me and the whole shop now knew it. Her voice was getting louder. "I want a new perm."

I looked over at my client who I had seen many

times and she looked at me as if to say—*Stand up for yourself, Kim.*

I wanted to reach across the front desk and punch trailer trash a few times to make it clear. No freebees unless you want a knuckle sandwich. But instead, I calmly told her that there is nothing I could help her with at this time.

The woman took her hot mess out the back door yelling. "You will hear from my lawyer." She got into her car. Her tires were throwing gravel everywhere as she raced out of the driveway.

My guest, who was now standing up and as angry as I was, told me how well I had handled the outburst. I was shaking with anger. I finished my day and wanted to just go home and take a long hot bath. I hoped that woman would never set foot in my shop again. Another good example why stupid should not reproduce. I felt so sorry for her little girl.

The next morning, the manager and I were opening and found that someone had egged our shop the previous night.

We were so mad, it took all our emotional energy we had to clean up the egg mess before clients began to arrive—there were at least a dozen raw eggs smeared on the front of my business.

I wonder who did it?

LESSONED LEARNED
You can't fix trailer trash stupid!

WE HAVE BEEN VANDALIZED

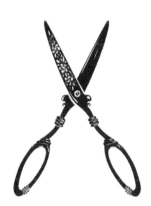

I made a pact with a friend and the deal worked out great... until...

I had been friends with John for a few years now. He wanted haircuts and I wanted my shop pressure washed once a year, so we decided to trade. I gave him a military man haircut once a month and he did the pressure washing of the entire building once a year.

One day, my manager called in a panic, "We have been tagged!"

I asked "What was tagged?"

Jewels, my manager said all the windows. I told her I would be right there. It was my Monday off, but as the owner I never really had a day off.

When I arrived, I saw the windows even before I drove into the driveway. They looked like someone had taken a shredder to each window screen. *What the fuck?*

I parked my car and got out in disbelief—thankfully the shop's siding looked clean and new. In contrast, the screens on the windows looked like someone had been very angry with them. I knew right then and there that it was my friend John. I called his number, I got his answering machine. I asked him to call me and before I could get out from behind the desk, John called me back.

"Signature Salon," I said, this is Kim. "John, did you happen to notice the screens—the shredded window screens?"

He said, "Yeah, but I did not do it on purpose."

I asked, "Did you notice what happened to the first screen after you hit it with the pressure washer stream? Why didn't you take off the other seven screens before washing?"

"I did not think I would hit a screen again," he said. "But I hit every one."

I said. "No shit!"

Needless to say, I replaced all the screens, and as far as John, we're still friends, I still cut his hair, but now he pays.

LESSON LEARNED

Friends and trading sometimes don't always work out. Make them pay instead!

SMURF BLUE

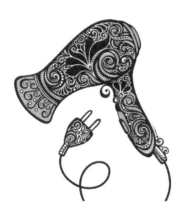

By this time I hired my first assistant. I had learned about her when she was working at a walk-in salon across town. She was pretty fresh out of Beauty College. I called her. "Hi, my name is Kim and I'm a salon owner looking for an assistant. I know you are at work so I will just leave my phone number. If you are interested call me." I said goodbye and in about ten minutes I got a call back when she was on a break. I told her what I was looking for in an assistant and she agreed to come in and check out my salon.

The day that she came, she was almost interviewing me; she was a few years older than me. She spent a full day in the waiting area, evaluating my salon and the people who worked with me. She seemed impressed. We got along very well. She started after she gave her two weeks' notice.

A young man, a college student, walked in. I sat

him at my station. My new assistant and I gave him a very good consultation and he told us he wanted to go BLUE! I was surprised! This was not the type of student I thought would want to go blue. He looked like a barber cut for sure and maybe even a pocket protector would be in order. He told us he wanted to stand out. *Okay!* My assistant was excited to get started.

I agreed that we would bleach this nineteen-year-old medium-brown head of hair to a pale yellow. He was surprised when he saw himself in the mirror. We then dried the hair and put on the intense blue. (Kind of a dark royal blue, like Smurf color.)

We educated him to be sure he knew that the first time he washed his hair he may find blue in his shower and to hang his head over and rinse so the blue would not stain his body.

I told him not to use a white towel due to the fact that it will stain the towel, too. He was so excited! He paid and gave my assistant, who did most of the work, a handsome tip. He grabbed his coat and walked out the front door. As I saw him walking to the bus stop, it started to rain. I could now see blue slightly running down his young face. I thought, *God, I hope the bus shows up soon or he will be a blue mess.*

I'm sure the bus driver was thinking… *Poor kid. Who did this to him? Is it a college prank?*

LESSON LEARNED
Some people like to stand out in a crowd.

REMEMBER ME?

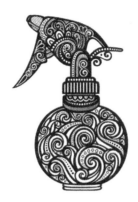

I had cut this woman's hair once before. As she walked into the salon, her Texas accent caught my attention as I was finishing the patron before her. She had not even made it to the waiting area before asking "Hi, remember me?"

I always greet people, but I wish they would have the common courtesy, when I have a guest in my chair, to wait until the conversation has a lull before interrupting. It's the person in the chair's appointment time. New arrivals should wait until they are acknowledged, as they arrive.

I replied "Yes, I remember you," thinking to myself that I wished I would have known it was her when she had made the appointment because she is a little "cray cray."

"I'll be with you in a few minutes. Would you like something to drink while you wait?" I said.

"I do have an appointment!" she said, almost condescending.

"Yes ma'am, you do have an appointment and it will start when I'm done with my client who is already in the chair!" Adding…"You do realize you are about fifteen minutes early?"

Oh," she said with a pouty face. I told her there were lots of books with haircuts in them, and if she wished, she could check them out. She was not interested in being patient, I could tell.

My guest in the chair was understanding about Miss Texas Drawl's impatience. She told me there was not a problem. I finished with her hair and she paid and was on her way.

I started to clean up my station, sweeping, but before I could get the dust pan down to pick up the hair, Miss Patience had placed her tiny, tight ass in my chair. She was an attractive woman—*if you like a horsey look.*

I went to the back room to put the towels in the washer and took a deep cleansing breath. One of my employees was grabbing her purse and told me she was going to lunch. That left me alone with Miss Patience—Miss Texas Drawl.

'Lo and behold' the phone rang. Not having a receptionist, I went straight to the phone answering, "Signature Salon, how can I help you?"

The woman on the other end was making appointments for the entire family: her two sons, her daughter and herself. This took a little bit of time and I could tell Texas Drawl was not happy with me.

I finished and went straight over to ask for forgiveness for taking up her precious time, even though her appointment time had not even started.

Everything seemed to be fine and I began to cut

her hair dry because that is what she requested me to do. The phone rang again and I excused myself and answered it, and another appointment was made.

I walked back over behind the chair—and I caught her using my shears, trying to cut her own hair! I told her, "I will take those please." She handed me the shears and I scolded her and told her these were my tools and I would prefer she not touch them. The phone rang again and I ignored it and let the answering machine get it this time.

Meanwhile, I was trying to fix what she had done to her hair with my shears while I was at the desk. The phone rang again and I still proceeded to work with this lady's hair. The bell went off at the door. I think, *Thank God.* Someone else to help, to distract me from little Miss Patience. It was a UPS man making a delivery. I signed my name, put the box in the back and came back to the station with Texan Drawl cutting her hair *again* with my shears.

I told her we were done and took the shears from her and the cape off of her. She asked if I was sure I had gotten it even. I told her "No, because you keep messing with it. If I came into your husband's work and took his tools (knowing her husband was a dentist of some sort) and began working on my own teeth, do you think he would let that happen or like it?"

"You wouldn't do that," she said. She did not think she had done anything wrong, even to this day I bet. (But lady you did. You messed with the wrong hairdresser!) She stood up on her tall horse and said "Well I guess I have to pay you?"

"Yes, yes, you do!"

She went into the hall towards the bathroom. She was so coo-coo for coco-puffs. She wanted her coat that was hung by the front desk, but she went the wrong direction in the salon. So I went to where her coat was and took it down and waited for her to figure out she was going the wrong way. I handed it to her and she paid and walked out the back door in a huff.

My employee, Mel, was coming back from lunch and got out of her car and got caught in her cross fire. "Kim just kicked me out of her salon!"

"What? That does not sound like Kim?" Mel, said. The woman got into her car and drove off with her tires squealing. Mel walked into the shop and wanted to know what the hell that was all about. I told her the story and she said "Wow, that has never happened to me before!"

"Me either, and I've been doing this for over ten years." But I guess you get new stories to tell every day when you work behind the chair.

LESSON LEARNED
Some women I will never undersand.

NBA

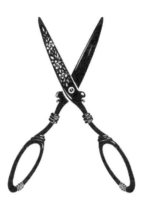

Nancy walked in for the first time. Nancy Butler Abbey, (called NBA for short), was now sitting in my chair. She had gone to a stylist in town that charged way too much for what she gave Nancy. Nancy told me how she had left the shop with pink, spiky-topped hair. I asked "Did you ask for pink hair?"

"NO!"

I was not keeping track, but I knew M.J. (My client that refers clients all the time) was doing me a huge favor. Each and every lady she sent into see me was a teacher or her friend. Great ladies in all.

I always ask where people work, or if they work from home as a domestic goddess, to help learn their hair needs and style. Nancy laughed with me, one of those welcoming laughs, fun and delightful, not obnoxious.

NBA told me she came over from the school where she worked across the street—and she had come through the bushes. So now she became the "Bush Woman" to me forevermore.

I colored her hair a beautiful shade of blonde and cut her hair to a reasonable, youthful length and got her out of the eighties, blending her spiky top with the lower half of her longer hair. I asked her, "So what did you do when the expensive salon on the other side of town turned your hair pink?"

She replied, "Well, I was shocked looking at myself in the mirror—and the stylist acted like it was wonderful!" She continued, "I walked out not paying, that's what happened, and the stylist had the gall to follow me outside and demand to be paid—so to avoid a scene, I paid!"

So, I guessed that the stylist really wanted to be a doctor, because even if they screw up, misdiagnose or botch a surgery they still get paid.

LESSON LEARNED
Paying more does not mean you get the best.

THE SALONS WINNING NAME

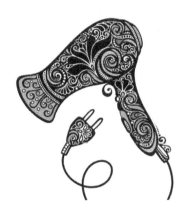

Shortly after I bought my salon, I had a contest to see if my clients could help me come up with a new business name. Never in a million years would I continue to call it Honeycomb. It's a hair salon not a cereal. It was originally called Pearl's House of Curls. Now that is a name! I was not willing to keep that original name either.

So... I had a glass bowl up at the front desk and told all the clients who walked in the door that I was running a contest for a new business name for my salon. The winner would receive a full makeover—a haircut, hair color, brow waxing, massage, facial, pedicure and manicure.

Several people entered the contest and we got lots of ideas that I would never, ever use. Some of my most memorable ones were: The Cat's Meow. What are we, a pet groomer? Another was, The Back Door Salon. Yes, most people come in through the back door due to the parking in the back, but this put me off—it sounded more like clients would get more than they bargained for. NO THANKS! The Phoenix was another suggestion: I did not know what that meant and thought others wouldn't either. (The bird that rises up from the fire and ash to renew youth, but what that has to do with a salon was lost on me.)

Then one day I was checking out a thick book while on a break in the back room. The book had salon pictures in it. It showed fronts of salons and ideas for interiors. One salon which was in another state had this cool logo and it read, "Signature Salon." It hit me just right. It sounded cool. I told a client about it who worked for a business office. She took it upon herself to suggest the name in my glass bowl, and she even went as far as to call to see if the name was taken as a business name in the State of Oregon registry.

On the tiny piece of off-white paper she wrote, "Signature Salon" along with a note that read, "The name is yours. I checked and you can even get a domain name." Winner! Winner! That is how I got my name for my salon. She was kind enough to go the extra mile and I paid her off with the best pampering of her life.

LESSON LEARNED
Everyone's tastes vary!

Lessons Learned Behind the Chair

IT'S OKAY TO DISCRIMINATE

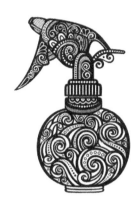

Hiring a new stylist is not as easy as you might think. I found that to be true in the late 1990s and early 2000s—when there was a shortage of good stylists who wanted to work.

I ran an ad in the local newspaper once. Never again! It was a waste of money. One woman called, and when I answered the phone, "Signature Salon, this is Kim how can I help you?" The voice on the other end said, "How much will I get paid?"

I said "Excuse me?"

The voice said again, "I'm calling about the ad in the paper. How much will I get paid?"

I stopped, dumbfounded that this so-called stylist was going to start out her inquiry about a job like this.

Taken aback, I responded as abruptly, "Probably nothing, because I wouldn't hire you." She was insulted.

Who starts out a conversation, on the phone, or otherwise, in their effort to get a job with, "How much will I make?" Most people ask about what the job entails to see if it's a good fit, and inquire about the employer's expectations, the hours, and then ask to come in to see the environment of the salon.

I told the voice on the phone that the amount a stylist makes is up to each one. If she or he is a team player and work hard, the sky is the limit. The voice on the other end went dead. I heard nothing. I said, "Hello," and still I heard nothing so I hung up.

I went back to what I was doing; folding towels in the back and then the phone rang again. I picked it up and started my spiel "Signature Salon…" and I was interrupted.

"I'm a team player!" the voice started in… "You don't know me, bitch!"

My heart started to pound as I stood in shocked silence, with the phone receiver in my hand—my mouth simply hung open, speechless for a few seconds. I was in disbelief of what she had just called me.

I took a second to breathe, and then the "pissed" kicked in.

"I don't believe you would fit in here," I said firmly. "You are not a team player and you definitely do not have any scruples or integrity, so I'm hanging up now and please do not call back. Good luck on finding a job with your interview skills—and holding on to a job with your manners—good day to you!"

I slammed the phone down and wanted to scream, "What is this world coming to?"

Not long after that *nondiscriminating job seeker*

call, Ellie, a young client who had just gotten married, told me she had a friend that was looking for a job doing hair.

I was excited and asked Ellie, "Is she normal? Ellie laughed and said "It depends."

I told Ellie to have her call me and we could get together to see if she would work out in my salon.

Kris walked in a week later for our first interview. She looked like she was in her 20s. She was not too tall—and she was very cute. She dressed like no other person, having her own style, but she *was normal!*

We talked, and I could tell she had been working in salons that were bigger and more chic. I explained that Signature is a family salon with four stations. (By now, the pink walls were all gone, and freshly painted white walls stood in their place.)

As we talked, I emphasized my cute, homey salon. I could tell she was interested and thinking about it. A day later she called and told me she would take the job.

Kris worked out great. Later I found out that she and her clients could speed talk—and when there were times that Kris was out and I took one of her clients on—I could not begin to keep up.

LESSON LEARNED
Speed talking is a talent, and I do not possess it!

Kimberly McBee

SISTERS

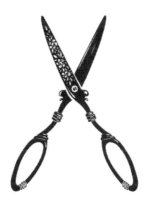

I have two sisters. One was eight years older, and one eight years younger than me. Yes, I'm the middle child. I'm sure when my older sister is being technical, she would say seven, but for being short one month I choose to say she is eight years older.

Some people say if you have a sister, your childhood is never lost. It's true!

I love them both. We are all three different in our own way and I thank God for that—in some ways more than others.

I thank my sisters for helping to make me who I am. I remember playing Barbies for days with my older sister. I forced my younger sister to play with us even though she would have rather have been outside throwing around a softball.

I have a vivid imagination due to the games I played as a child. Those poor Barbies, as you can imagine, all got haircuts. My sisters were willing to be models for me when I wanted to pretend and practice with hair when I was a teen, and also when I was in Beauty College.

Sorry Keri, for making you look like the Bride of Frankenstein in the sixth grade. Forgive me?

LESSON LEARNED
Never frost anyone's hair before you know what you are doing!

SOME HIDEOUS HIRING

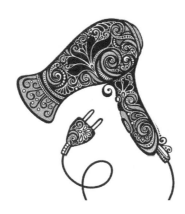

I interviewed many women over the years—some hideous, some not. One young woman I interviewed was fresh out of Beauty College. She was full of energy and did pedicures and manicures and artificial nails. She was such a hard worker and people loved her. But when cheap nail salons started up and took business from her, she left. I was sorry to lose her.

I hired a woman going into menopause and she put out a hit on each client she worked on. I was scared of her, she would switch personalities in seconds, nice one second and frantic the next. When one client came to me and told me she frightened her, and asked me to never schedule her with her again, I stopped giving her clients altogether. She left.

Next one I hired, I decided I had hired a psycho. When I talked to her, her eyes would shift to the right. She spent five hours on one set of nails and they looked like hell. She lasted two days. I began to ask people I planned to hire to bring in a model so I could see their work. Live and learn.

Thankfully, for ten years I had a really good crew. My manager, Jewels, was a wonderful business person and the clients loved her. During that time we had ten women working with us, some job sharing. Many were moms that wanted to spend time with their family and still come home with a paycheck.

LESSON LEARNED
Work smarter not harder!

OUR MADDI SURPRISE

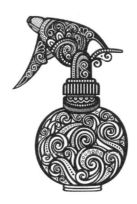

By this time, I had been married ten years. Where had the time gone? Mark and I were repeatedly told, "No babies." We were unable to conceive a baby—at least that had been true for over ten years.

We did our best to accept it, and worked to make other dreams come true. We bought the salon and the new house and thought, "This is our life." The salon was doing well. Three years in, and we had changed it for the better, and that felt great. There were no more Pepto-Bismo pink walls and no more artificial flowers. I was happy with how I had upgraded it, and we now had a full house.

It was then that the surprising news came. I bought a home pregnancy test kit and peed on the stick. It was a plus sign. What the hell! For real?

I showed the white stick to Mark, and yes, he confirmed it was a *plus sign,* plain as day. "Go to the doctor," he said. I felt a little weight that did not feel normal. I thought I had a tumor. Cancer? I went to the doc and he confirmed it—we were pregnant. Holy cow!

Okay, now what? The salon was going strong and the women working it were wonderful. And me? I was going to have a baby...

LESSON LEARNED

This was the best gift that could have ever been given to me.

BIG NEWS TO TELL MY FAMILY

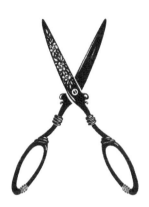

I couldn't wait to share this life-changing news!

I called my mother and asked if she and my stepfather could meet me for lunch. They were able to meet me at a cute place that in the 1950s was a filling station. Now it was a diner full of antiques from that era.

We were seated in the middle of the restaurant, on little red chairs. I was so excited to tell my secret. I was sitting across the table from them, and will never forget my mother's face when I told her I was going to make her a grandmother. She did have four grandchildren already, but since we did not think having children was possible, she cried tears through her smiling face. Not the ugly cry of someone in pain, but the tears of a person who is so happy for an especially joyous occasion.

My step-father never cried, but he was very happy about it; I could tell. I wasn't his own blood, but he always treated me as his own. They had married when I was five.

After nine months of feeling great and only gaining nineteen pounds, I gave birth to a perfect baby—a blue-eyed bald beauty. She had a small dimple on the left side of her face. My mother alway's said that she was kissed by an angel.

We named her Madison Nicole McBee... I wanted her initials to be MNM.

LESSON LEARNED
Babies are hard work!

SECOND SURPRISE

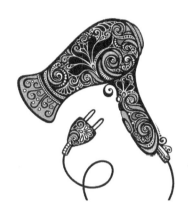

I went to the Beauty College to get a pedicure, so that I could meet (and hire) a young woman named Chrissy. I had my little Maddi in her car carrier and walked in with my skanky toes that had not been touched since before I went in to delivery.

I was greeted by the front desk student and lots of old memories came flooding back. I had not set foot in the Beauty College since the day I graduated, more than ten years before.

She told me to have a seat and before I could set the baby carrier down a young brunette called my name. I followed her, watching, as she had a skip in her step. She was not tall at all, but I didn't want to call her short. But she was maybe only five feet tall. Chrissy was very cute.

She had me sit down. Towels were on the floor next to an old looking plastic tub filled with soapy water. She asked me to place my feet in the tub since I had already taken my shoes off. I was wearing shorts. Baby Maddi was asleep in her carrier.

Chrissy commented on her, saying she had never seen such a beautiful baby. Obviously this was scoring points. She gave me a very nice pedicure and I told her why I was really there. We talked about her coming to work for Signature Salon and doing hair and nails, as an apprentice.

She hugged me and was so excited for this opportunity. She became a wonderful asset to my shop. Years later she was involved with a young man and thought she would marry him. She then decided that he was not her prince on the white horse after all. He decided to move to another state and she stayed put. One day after his move, Chrissy found out she was pregnant.

Pursuing education while being a hair stylist is not required, however, to be a better stylist/salon owner it is ideal to keep up on current trends and learn new techniques. So… I thought… *Vegas has one of the biggest hair shows, let's go to Vegas, baby!*

The salon was going and whoever could go, I wanted to join me. Chrissy, being early in her pregnancy was able to go, no problem. My first apprentice had never been to Vegas, so I really wanted her to go. Of course she was told "whatever happens in Vegas stays in Vegas." I rented a limo to pick us all up and drive us down the Vegas strip. That was a memory, to watch grown women hang out the moon roof and act like women gone wild.

My husband went to Vegas, too, so that he could golf with his brother, but I think it really was to keep all of us girls out of trouble. We took every class we could. Paul Mitchell was on stage. Redken was coloring plum red then. Extensions were the newest thing, glueing in wefts of hair, while not giving any thought to the abuse it causes to the natural hair.

At dinner at "The House of Blues," Chrissy was not ordering any alcoholic beverages. I told her I would not drink either. "Who knew that I could be pregnant, too?" We all laughed about that later, because little did I know at the time.

We went out to a casino after dinner and I was on a "Wheel of Fortune" machine, and everyone else was nowhere to be seen. I hit a three-hundred dollar jackpot. I was so excited that the woman next to me and I were hugging.

I fought my way through the New York, New York Casino, and I spotted Mark, the other girls, and his brother. I excitedly told them my fabulous news, but they were already celebrating.

Chrissy had just won fifteen-hundred dollars on a Wheel of Fortune machine. I slid my measly three-hundred dollars in my pocket and said, "Dinner's on you!"

Later that night, after walking the full Vegas strip, the girls talked me into getting a pregnancy test. Again, I was so surprised to see the plus sign… Yes, again!

The moral of the story: ten years for the first baby and only thirteen months for the second…

LESSON LEARNED
Doctors don't know everything.

Kimberly McBee

ADVERTISING

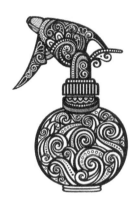

I tried it all, but referrals by word-of-mouth are still the proven best: Back then, I did try the newspaper. Not worth it. The ad man I was working with did not get me. He came in with a mock-up of an ad that looked like it was from the 1950s. He had a woman dressed in an apron peeking into the ad. "Hell no mister," I told him.

    I tried radio, and it was fun to hear the ad, but I don't think I ran it often enough and it was expensive. Next came T.V. Commercials—that really was fun. We did before and after looks on three lovely ladies. We had music and shots of the salon on the inside and out. The ad showed us in action. I was excited to include Maddi's face on T.V. at age two. This would show that we served all ages. It was then that I got my first clue into the challenges of motherhood—she refused and was never in the commercial.

    I was happy that we did get a lot of response

from the T.V. Commercial. We ran it right before the five o'clock news and after the Oprah Winfrey show. Lots of people saw it. I don't know how well commercials work today, with DVR's, and everyone speeding through the commercials after recording their shows. Maybe not so good.

LESSON LEARNED
Word-of-mouth costs nothing. At the same time, positively selling yourself and your skills—that's the key to good marketing.

Lessons Learned Behind the Chair

THAT ONE CLIENT

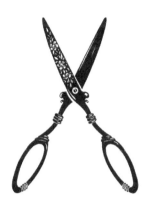

There is always one! Yes, there is that one male client that comes in and all the stylists act like they are in heat. With this one client, when he walked in, one of the stylists hid out in the back room, due to the scent of his testosterone that seemed to seep out of his pores. One stylist turned bright red and acted like a little girl who has never been kissed. Another stylist flaunted herself as if to giggle uncontrollably, while showing some cleavage.

This "one client's" name was Thomas. He walked in for the haircut he had scheduled every three weeks, like clockwork.

"Hello Kimberly," he would say while seating himself, waiting for his turn. I welcomed him and could already smell his fragrance. I bent to sweep the hair off the floor as I do many times a day, but this time I take careful measure to look like a lady. I bent my knees to the side, so as not to stick my big ass in the air. The massage therapist walked out from the back so her client could disrobe. I noticed that she took an awfully long time to let her client get comfortable, face down on the massage bed. She spent the time flirting with Mr. Handsome. She was not afraid of pretty men. In fact, I saw her undressing him with her eyes. She never got the pleasure of massaging his beautiful tan muscles, but I have a feeling she would not stop at his biceps.

I called Thomas over. "I'm ready for you." His smile just melted me; it left me feeling like putty. He sat down and I put the black silk-like drape around his beautiful neck. There is something about a man's neck. I love the look of the strong, sculpted hairline of a man's neck… hmm….

He looked into my eyes through the reflection in the mirror, and I could see the twinkle he always had when he looked at me. Maybe he did this with every woman, but I wanted to think it was just for me. I had cut his hair for years, and when I first started several years before, I would break out into a sweat. I stuttered, making a total fool of myself, but he always seemed to be flattered by this. I think it was not uncommon for women to act unusual in his presence.

I cut his hair as I always did, and in three weeks there was not a huge amount of hair to cut, but I took my time, just to spend more time talking to him. I could tell he was a hardworking man and a good soul. When I was finished, we walked to the desk and all the women scattered. He paid and I rescheduled him for the next appointment three weeks after this one. As he walked out the door, I thought once again, "Only three weeks until I get this high again."

LESSON LEARNED

I'm a married woman. I'm a married woman, and oh yes, he's a married man. He is a married man!

Kimberly McBee

BIKINI WAXING EXTRAORDINAIRE

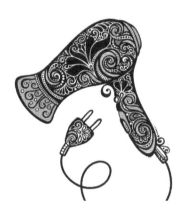

I was trained in waxing. I guess I don't mind inflicting pain on people for some strange reason. I have no feeling that I'm hurting them by putting sweet smelling, warm, honey based wax on their skin—as I help them to get rid of the hair that they do not wish to keep.

One afternoon I knew I had a bikini wax appointment scheduled after lunch. I prepped the back room for the service, which included fresh sheets on the massage/facial/waxing table. I turned on soft music and lit a comforting smelling candle.

I greeted the average height soccer mom with her bountiful red hair. I led her to the back room and asked if she would like any beverage. She said, "I just had lunch, so thanks, but no thanks."

I had her sit down on the high wing back chair. I asked if she had ever had this waxing done before. She said "No!" I told her what to expect. I explained that she would need to disrobe from the waist down, but could leave her socks on. I left a fresh starched sheet for her to cover herself.

The room smelled sweet when I left to wash my hands in the restroom across the hall. I went back to the door and tapped, asking softly if she was ready. I heard her jump on the bed as she said with a stressed voice "Yes!" I could hear that she was uncomfortable.

I entered the low lit room. She was lying flat on her back, with the sheet pulled up to her chin. I explained that I would be lifting the sheet and I would do one side at a time, and only one leg would be exposed. I told her that I would apply a numbing agent first.

Little did I know that *I didn't know what to expect.* I lifted the sheet and slid it to expose the biggest bush I have ever seen. She was not only red upstairs, but the downstairs was fiery red also. *The carpet matched the drapes,* as they say. I talked to her about shape, while waiting the full thirty seconds that it takes for the numbing to take effect.

I excused myself and went out to get the hedge trimmer—I mean to grab the hair trimmer and attachments to tame this red, curly beast. When I returned to the room she had relaxed. I lifted the sheet once again. Even the second time I was surprised by the mass. I told her I was going to shorten it up some before I applied any wax. I could not see any skin. I took the handheld cordless clippers that are rechargeable. I was glad they had the full charge, because I was going to need it.

I trimmed seven times with different length attachments to get down to the average person's pubes. I spent fifteen minutes and by then the numbing was wearing off. I re-applied the numbing agent on both sides and waited the time needed. I applied my first thin layer of wax on her pale inner thigh. I placed the waxing paper and gave my first pull. She almost came off the table. Her hair was so deep rooted that I knew that this was harder on her than on me. I put pressure from my full palm and pressed. She was in instant relief.

The next layer of wax went on between the top of her patch and hip bone and once again I pulled. Not as traumatic. The next layer was going on the bottom of the patch to remove the curly red short pubes. Now this was going to hurt. I put my arm strength to work and pulled.

Tears were forming and I saw a path starting to trickle down her face. I hoped she could fight through the pain. For her first time at this, she was doing pretty well; she was not yelling. I finished two hours later.

Normal bikini waxing takes forty minutes to an hour. This was not normal.

LESSON LEARNED
I'll never go native and no one else should either.

Kimberly McBee

HAIR SHOW LET DOWN

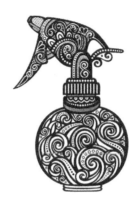

Branches? Branches in the hair style? *What's this?* It didn't take long to wish we had been "no shows" at this out-of-state Seattle hair show.

Why did we pay good money for this fiasco? There we sat stiffly in uncomfortable folding chairs at the conference, watching the platform artist make volunteer model's hair into some sort of tree. All the time, they played obnoxiously loud music and made us dizzy with fancy lights.

The platform artist dramatically cut, styled and tortured these poor individuals on stage to impress the audience of hairstylists. We all watched intently, hoping to take back information on new trends and creative ideas. Nope, not this time. For sure, I have never—and will never—put branches in my client's hair.

My clients would not pay for that style or service. I have seen some pretty outrageous creations. I had gone to this Seattle show wanting to learn a new haircut or color technique for my salon knowledge—not learn landscaping techniques.

LESSON LEARNED

On second thought—I could have used landscaping lessons for my bikini waxing!

BROWS FRAME THE FACE

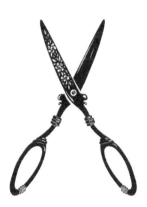

I was about to grab my lunch from the fridge when a young lady walked in and asked for a brow waxing. I took a good look at her; she was gorgeous.

Why not? I thought. *I will eat later.*

I prepped the shampoo bowl where I waxed eyebrows. I made her comfortable with a soft white towel behind her neck as she leaned back on the bowl.

I combed her hair, putting in clips, so it stayed out of the way. Then I discovered she only had one eyebrow.

I sold her an eyebrow pencil.

LESSON LEARNED
Don't let your sister wax your brows.

Kimberly McBee

Lessons Learned Behind the Chair

GOING FROM NEW TO OLD

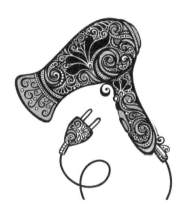

It was really a sunny day—Mark and I were enjoying our drive around the country neighborhood. Both kids were sound asleep in their car seats. Checking out a garage sale is what we thought we were doing out there—we had not planned on finding a new home. We saw a for sale sign that read, "Shop for Sale." I immediately asked him to stop.

He said to me, "Let's just call the number."

I almost yelled for him to stop the car. He was so startled; he did what I was pleading him to do.

He rolled to a stop and I stepped right out of the car and walked up to knock on the front door. A young woman, about my age, opened the door. Behind her I can see a naked little girl running around.

She apologized. "We are potty training our youngest." The little girl is the same age as my son, Jack, so I completely understood.

I asked if we could see the place, or if we should call the realtor instead? The woman said, "Sure, just come on in."

I waved to Mark, who is now looking at me with a pleading face to leave. He parked the truck in the shade, with the kids sound asleep. He got out of the truck, unwillingly.

As we took a quick look, the woman apologized again, this time for the dirty clothes on the laundry room floor. I reminded her, "Hey, we came in on you unexpectedly. No need to apologize."

We saw the front room with floor to ceiling windows. The windows looked out onto the back yard which we thought was beautiful. The property is two acres. *I'm sold!*

In the back, the woman's mother and husband were in the raspberry patch picking berries, and the two young girls were on the tire swing that hung from the huge cherry tree. I could see us making similar memories on this land.

Mark and I made an offer on this 1950s ranch style home and got the house. We sold our newer home in three days. It must be a trend for us to sell houses so fast. It was a little hard to go from a brand new house to an older style, but it was so worth the struggles of time spent remodeling.

LESSON LEARNED
A little piece of heaven sometimes calls your name.

BIG BOY PANTS

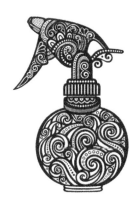

Our son Jack was almost three when he started to wear "big boy pants." He was very proud of the fact that he wasn't in diapers anymore. Needless to say, it made me pretty happy too!

One night, we met my family at a local seafood restaurant for dinner. While waiting for our table, we sat in the lobby with the other guests. Jack proudly began to tell his Grandpa Lynn about his new Spiderman big boy pants.

Grandpa paid close attention, telling him "That's great; I'm very proud of you!"

About that time, Jack decided to show Grandpa and the world. He yanked his britches to his ankles to show off his Spiderman underwear. An older man sitting next to Dad howled in laughter as Jack *showed off* his underwear, stating in his toddler voice, "These are great big boy pants!"

LESSON LEARNED

If you've got it, flaunt it!

POOP-POTPOURRI

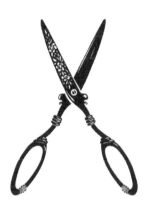

I was cutting a fireman's hair. My son's daycare was on vacation, so he was spending the afternoon at the salon. I had a DVD of Scooby-Doo to keep him occupied while I finished my work behind the chair.

The salon had a room for massage, but the massage therapist was done for the day. So I had the little man set up with snacks and a pillow and blanket. I saw him go into the bathroom. At three, he had just started to wear big boy pants. I continued cutting the middle-aged man's hair. Then I saw my son come out with tears—and he began to scream.

Poor little man. His pants were undone and his zipper was totally unzipped. I dropped my shears and comb on the counter. I left the undone haircut and grabbed my son and took him back into the bathroom—concerned that he had zipped his penis into his zipper. *No, thank goodness, it was still totally attached!*

But he was still screaming bloody murder! What had he done? I stripped him and saw his whole genital area was flaming red.

"What did you put on little man? Did you wash with soap?"

He pointed at the orange deodorant room spray. He said. "I'm sorry, mommy, I'm sorry, mommy" He kept saying it over and over. I felt like the people out in the salon probably thought I was beating him.

I filled the sink and I set his stripped bare bottom in the cool water. He stopped screaming and apologizing—and let out a huge sigh of relief... The spray had burned his sack. Poor little dude.

He said, "I just wanted to smell good!" I smiled and hugged him.

I got him happily settled back in with a cozy blanket and Scooby Doo, then went back to finish my client's hair. He acted like nothing had happened. Not one comment or question. Evidently, he only wanted to get his cut done so he could leave.

Me? I was stressed!

LESSON LEARNED

"It's all about me" is a good analogy for some people.

MY MOTHER – GOD REST HER SOUL

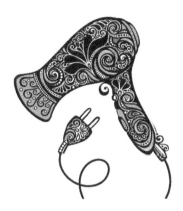

My mother came in for a party-do. She was going to have me shampoo and style her hair. She needed to use the restroom. After I shampooed her hair, she headed into the powder room.

My mother returned and sat in the chair so I could begin to blow dry her wet hair. She kept wiggling around—she was almost dancing in the chair.

I told her it was not easy to style her hair while she was moving so much. She wiggled and wiggled. I finally finished, trying not to burn her with the curling iron. She told me later that she had taken that orange deodorant, room spray and sprayed her privates.

Really, Mom? It must be genetic! Of course it burned her too. Why, at over sixty years old, in God's name, would she spray her most tender body parts with orange air spray for household odors? Who does that?

She did. She wanted to smell good.

LESSON LEARNED
Oranges do not fall far from the tree.

LOSS

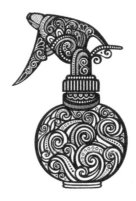

One day while working behind the chair, the phone rang and it was my stepfather. He told me that my mother was not able to get up. I told him that I would be there as soon as I could. I was in the middle of cutting a client's hair, so I asked one of the girls to take over for me.

When I arrived at my parents home, my father had already had left—he had gone ahead and driven himself to an appointment for a chemo treatment. He had been diagnosed with cancer not too long before this.

I helped my mother up. He could not do it, because he was very weak from his ongoing chemo treatments.

At the time, I felt that she may have had a stroke. I got her an appointment with her doctor for the next day.

It went down hill from there. She was admitted to the hospital for a stroke, then she moved to rehab—

but during that short three-week period, she was diagnosed with cancer herself. Her health quickly went from bad to worse when they found her liver riddled with cancer. Me and my family were devastated.

The doctor's told us that the time she had was limited—only days or weeks left. Shocking! We put all our efforts into getting her back home as soon as possible—and thankfully, we were able to get her home the next evening.

She passed that night. I thank God we got her home and her children were with her. She was only sixty-nine years of age—cancer sucks!

After my mother passed in February, in October we lost my stepfather. These losses were the hardest experiences of my life.

God bless my parents for my childhood.

LESSON LEARNED
Don't take people for granted, they may not always be here.

SIGNATURE SALON

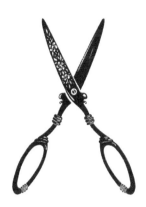

All good things must come to an end. After owning the salon for eleven years, it was time for a change.

I hope all the girls in the salon who were employed by me, or leased from me, know how dear they all still are to me. That was a season when I was under a lot of stress with the kids getting older, and stylists moving on—I did not have the energy to start over with a new crew.

Jewels had built a salon on the side of her home and others had either moved away or started their own salons.

I decided it was time to call it quits in this venue, so I sold the little 1930's house/salon. As usual, my instinct and timing was right—I found a buyer really fast. I sold, but gave the women who worked for me one full year's notice so they could figure out their next adventure.

My husband, Mark, remodeled our one car garage and made a beautiful hair studio for me.

LESSON LEARNED
Something old and ugly can turn out pretty darn sweet!

ADDITION

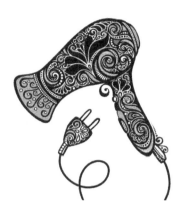

Have you ever done a DIY remodel? We have, more than once! My studio, converted beautifully into a hair studio—the former garage space—long gone!

A real plus is that it now has two huge windows. One in the front to see into the studio and one the same size on the opposite end, next to my station. If you stand out in front of the studio you can look through the window and into the backyard. I take a lot of pride in our yard. Maybe not as much as my lovely husband, who loves to mow the grass two times a week and make everything look pretty, but it sure is nice to hear my clients compliment the view—it is a relaxing and peaceful environment for them as they sit in the chair.

We removed twenty-six trees from the backyard, and there are still two dozen trees, of all types, in the back acreage.

When we completed the remodel, we had an

open house to show my clientele that I would not be shampooing their heads in the kitchen sink! The wood mahogany floors looked great, up against walls painted a soft beige with Merlot colored curtains. I also painted white trim on the windows.

The shelves and desk are mahogany, leaning and tethered to the wall. I have a wine cabinet and a small fridge to offer clients a cold beverage.

There is a comfortable leather couch against one wall and two leather chairs in the waiting area. I have music playing, and the clients smell a clove candle by Loma as they walk in the door. I love this scent. It has something to do with my childhood memories.

I feel as if I get to experience the best of both worlds. I offer my clients a welcoming, comfortable space. I get to continue offering my professional best, and I also get to be a mom that is home for my school-age kids.

I simply have to walk from my hair studio through a door to the entry and utility area—then take two steps through the opposite door to get into my home. So as you can see from a business perspective it is a totally separate space, but from my family's perspective, I can always be there for them. This addition is much more than it appears on the surface!

LESSON LEARNED
Sometimes you are put in a place where you are absolutely meant to be.

BUSH MAN

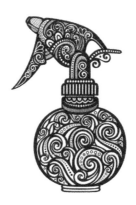

Working from my salon on the side of the house, my first client of the day is one lady whom I love. Nancy—and she is funny and full of life. As I finished foiling her head with blonde highlights, suddenly the neighbor girl comes in all scared looking. "There is a guy in your bushes?"

I walked out, adorned with my color-soaked gloves and apron, where I saw a man in the bushes on the side of my garage. "Can I help you?" I asked.

"I'm just getting out of the rain," he responded. He looked creepy, so I pulled out my confident, commanding mom voice. I told him, "Keep moving." I believed he was peeping on the young, pretty neighbor girl.

When I finished with Nancy in my chair, she was willing to go out and drive by in her car to make sure this Peeping Bush Man was gone. No sign of him...

LESSON LEARNED
Don't mess with a hairdresser in the middle of coloring someone's hair!

GOOD HEAD

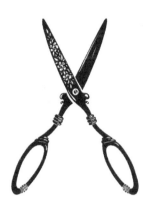

Shampooing a client's hair can and should be a great experience for the client. When I'm shampooing someone and they start to moan it can get uncomfortable. Some stylists can take it as a compliment I suppose.

As one woman was leaning back to get her brows waxed, she told me she did not want a shampoo with her trim. "Not that you don't give good head." She turned red immediately.

I could not contain myself—I laughed out loud. She quickly restated it to make herself clear. "I mean you give a good shampoo."

"I know what you mean," I told her. It made my day. I love to laugh, and that sure gave me a good laugh.

I guess that goes along with a woman asking for a blow job. I asked her again, "So you want a shampoo and blow dry?" It was a little surprising to me when she repeated in this way—"I would like to get a blow job."

No pun intended, but I was blown away when she said that! My thoughts went every-which-way. *Sure, we give the best blowjobs in town. Come on in and have a seat. Let me get the best blowjob expert I know—and get her right out here for you.*

I went into the back room where a new stylist was sitting, waiting for her next opportunity to have a butt in her chair.

"There is a new client that just walked in and asked for a blow job." I told her you are the best in town, so she is waiting."

The expression on the newbie's face was priceless. "What does she want me to do?"

"Shampoo and blow dry, but I'm warning you, she call's it a blow job."

LESSON LEARNED
People say the funniest things.

WHEN THE COW COMES HOME

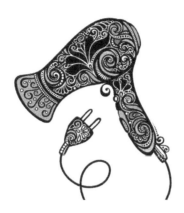

Connie was leaning back in the shampoo bowl, and loving the shampoo I was providing for her. My daughter walked into the salon. She had been mowing the lawn on the John Deere riding mower a minute before, and now was standing in the doorway, hysterical. My first thought was that she had hurt herself. Maybe she had cut off a finger or run over one of our wiener dogs. Maddi looked like she had all her fingers and toes, but she was crying, red faced—and she could barely talk.

I got her to calm down long enough to tell me that while giving the lawn clippings to the neighbor's cows, the little black calf had escaped. We live on the edge of town and the neighbors have cows, but it's not like we live in the middle of nowhere. A calf wandering into the street or another neighbor's yard could create some problems.

Feeding the fat cows made them happy, so we shared our clippings with them, and then we didn't have to pay to dispose of them either.

Back to the story: So Maddi had let one of the cows escape, and Connie was still hanging in the shampoo bowl and my hands were covered in suds. I excused myself from shampooing. Connie was okay with me leaving the conditioner on her hair for a few minutes.

I went out in my work attire, which by the way isn't farm friendly. With my color apron on and shoes not meant for running, I ran across the freshly mown grass. Maddi was running behind me and not helping—since she still was crying and had tears streaming down her face.

I told her to drive the mower in to block in such a way that the cow could not go around it. Then the cow started to head towards the main road. *I panicked!*

I went into the other neighbor's yard, running in my wedged heels and looked over to see the neighbor lady peering out her window. She had to be wondering why I was running along her fence line; so I waved and smiled. *Just a normal day in the life of Kim!*

I still looked like I was ready to color someone's hair. Mind you, during this time, the cow is heading down the gravel driveway to the main road. I managed to come through the fence right in front of the cow, and we had a stand off.

The cow looked at me and I looked at the cow. I started to run towards it and the cow backed down and ran in the other direction. Maddi and the John Deere were in front of the gate that leads back into the five acres where the other cows were watching us—probably thinking—*fools!*

My efforts finally got the young black calf back in where she was supposed to be, where she happily started eating the remains of the grass clippings.

I had worked up quite a sweat and started heading back to the salon with Maddi. I put my arm around my tear-streaked daughter and told her how much I loved her, and we both laughed. Today, we retell this story when we need a good laugh.

LESSON LEARNED

I can outrun a cow while doing hair and consoling my freaked out daughter. I also found out from the neighbor that the cow's name was "Sneaky."

Kimberly McBee

TWENTY YEARS

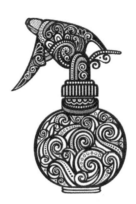

Married for twenty years. WOW, how and when did that happen? Maybe I fell asleep some time ago and just woke up. I swear it feels like yesterday when I was newly married wondering what life had in store for us.

We have been through so much of life together. Me working for some interesting people, to evolving into becoming my own boss Then after being the boss for many years, I now enjoy being on my own, knowing I only have to worry about me. My life, I have to say has been a blessing. Two kids and a wonderful and supportive husband.

Speaking of my husband. This year it was his turn. Each year we trade off. One year I plan what we do on our anniversary and he plans the next. He told me to take the time off for ten days and we would do something special. I could not contain myself. I love and hate surprises. I wanted to know what we would be doing, so Mark told me to guess, and if I guessed where we're going, he would tell me.

I start guessing. "Hawaii?"

"No," he said.

"Cancun?" I whispered.

"No."

I guessed a million places: Jamaica, Florida Keys, or Europe? No, No, No!

I was about to give up all my guessing, when one day while I was working the mailman came. I went out to get the mail. In the mailbox there was a letter and it was from a travel agent. I took it into the house and went back into the salon to prep for the next client. It was killing me, I wanted to open it. I saw my client drive in and while I cut her hair into a cute little stacked bob, I was thinking *I should not open that letter.*

Next thing I knew the client was leaving in her car and I was left alone with the letter. You guessed it; I opened the letter. Yes, it was from the travel agent and our flight had been changed—just a small five minute delay. *Why did they send a letter for that?*

I see our destination written right there—I'm going to the Cook Islands! Okay, but where the hell was that? Rarotonga to be exact. I sort of knew where to guess where it was, but where in the flipping world is Rarotonga?

I grabbed my globe that was sitting on my computer desk and looked and looked, and still did not see it anywhere. After I had stared at it forever, I finally saw a spec at the bottom of the South Pacific.

The Cook Islands and Rarotonga are close to New Zealand. How in the world did Mark decide on that place?

Mark came home and I started in while making dinner. Was it Italy, or was it New Zealand? Australia? I saw the *"you're getting hot"* look on his face. Is it Rarotonga?

He looked so disappointed. I had destroyed the surprise. I felt bad for about a split second. Then I jumped up and down since I knew where we were going. I showed him the letter and then the shit hit the fan.

After calling *to chat* with the travel agent, who was not supposed to send anything home, my husband got a few extra perks for us: we were booked first class and got a hiking outing with one of the natives, and our anniversary dinner, all compliments from the travel agency. I should have felt bad for the ass chewing the travel agent got, but we got a first class baby...

LESSON LEARNED
Being a brat has always paid off. *Why stop now?*

Kimberly McBee

FURRY FRIENDS

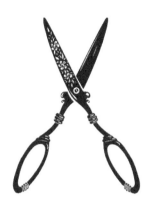

Sally, a regular client, walked in with the stroller in front of her. Most people would think she was rolling a baby in to the salon, but it was her furry friend. NBA, Nancy, is getting her hair foiled. I looked up and greeted Sally with a friendly, "Hello, I'll be with you soon."

She replied, "I know I'm early. While waiting, Sally takes her puppy out of the stroller and begins playing with the little guy. She had walked him before coming into the studio.

NBA turned and was facing the two on the couch: the puppy was enjoying the freedom out of the stroller. Before I knew what was happening NBA says in a loud, shocked tone of voice—"Is she wiping that dog's butt?"

I turned to see Sally cleaning the dog's behind with a tissue. I did not know what to say; I was speechless as NBA waited for me to answer.

I pretended to be blind, deaf and mute—I did not

see, nor did I hear a question. I *do not* love being put in these type of situations. You tell me—would you reply?

Lesson Learned
Sometimes being *behind the chair* can be the shits.

DOGGIES

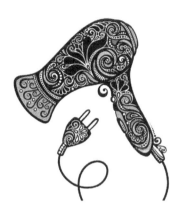

When we moved the salon into my home, we had a 147 pound black lab, named Riley. Everybody loved Riley. He was a smart dog. We had an invisible fence that made him stay in the yard; he had two acres to roam. He gently greeted all my clients as they walked in. Like I said, everybody loved Riley. Early one morning he wanted to go out. We let Riley out around three in the morning. We did not know he had found a glitch in the invisible fence.

A client who walked in the early mornings came in later, and she told me that an animal had come out of the bushes that morning while she was walking—she thought it was a bear. She was scared. *Maybe something else?*

We talked and decided Riley must have gotten out. But no way—Riley, aka Mr. Smarty Pants, stayed all day long in the yard greeting clients, sleeping in his favorite spot and then at three in the morning he wanted outside. He repeated that pattern day-after-day.

Okay, maybe today was different. I thought he was just a hot dog and want to cool off. So... truth be told, Riley *had* figured out how to cruise the neighborhood and swim in the neighbors' ponds, and also visit other dogs that slept outside. Quite the roundabout.

We fixed the fence and he did not "bear scare" any other early morning walkers.

RIP Mr. Riley. Love you forever.

LESSON LEARNED
Dogs are great friends!

HEY KID

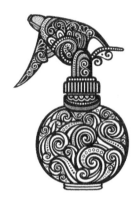

As you know, I have a lot of teachers as clients. One of my sweet, redheaded retired clients referred a new butt to sit in my chair. She walked in, and she was also a retired teacher.

"Hey kid," she said, while she introduced herself. I said "Hello." I was still finishing the client before her. She was a little early and I asked if she would like to sit in the massage chair.

Immediately, I knew I was going to like her. She sat in the massage chair and made relaxed humming sounds, because she liked the way the massage felt on her back. She cracked both me and my other client up. When I was done, my current client paid and walked out the door.

I interrupt my humming guest from her massage and said, "Come on down. You're the next contestant!"

She smiled and headed to the station. While behind the chair I analyzed her hair and her face shape and body style. She was very pretty and took good care of herself, even though she and her friends tended to be so hard on themselves.

You know, as women, I believe we are our own worst enemy when it comes to staring at ourselves in the mirror. If I were able to tell all my clients what I truly think of them, they would see themselves in the mirror as I do. If so, they would think they were drop dead gorgeous. Personality and being a good person is much more attractive than some of the people that could be (or are) on the front page of a magazine.

Now, tell me how you could not just love a person who every time they walked into the studio said, "Hey Kid!"

LESSON LEARNED
Become more like the people I admire.

TWENTY-FIVE YEARS

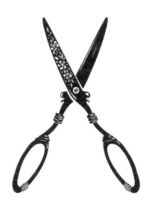

As I'm finishing this book, we have been married twenty-five years. Hmm…

Hey, we are still talking! The kids are growing up and my salon is still going strong. It's my year, my turn, to plan the trip.

I have a beautiful lady client, Mary Jane, who owns a home not too far from me and one in the Cayman Islands. For the last ten years she has tried to get me to come visit and stay with them at their home there.

Finally, this year, I talked to Mary Jane and told her my husband and I could come if she would have us. She was so excited. It made us feel even better about going. I knew it would be fun.

We flew out and it took a long time. With my husband traveling for work, he has a lot of flight miles, so that's how we are able to travel more, but sometimes when using mileage it's a roundabout way. We took six flights before reaching our destination. We got off the plane and Mary Jane and her husband were waiting for us, waving—and in excited voices saying "Hello McBee's..."

We got our luggage and headed to the parking lot. With the steering wheel on the opposite side of the car, it was different, but we all got in. Before the wheels of the car even started turning, Mary Jane pulled out the pineapple juice and coconut rum! Let's get this party started, was all I could think. I could not see straight by the time we reached their cute little bungalow.

It was two stories and right on the beach. I mean we stepped out and it was literally eight steps to the water. We headed to our space and put our bags in the upstairs room with a bath reserved for us. It has two single beds... I start to laugh! Happy anniversary, honey.

The weather was nice and sunny, and the ocean was blue like a picture postcard. We made plans to go snorkeling the next day. While getting ready for the snorkel trip, we discovered the kids had taken out our goggles. We had the snorkel mouth piece and the snorkel fins, but no goggles. M.J. came to the rescue. She loaned us each a pair and we headed out.

Her husband dropped us all off at the snorkel sight after leaving a car at Rum Point where we would be snorkeling to... *I love saying snorkel don't you?*

We were barefoot and ready to get into the water. Then Mark and I noticed that neither of us have our clip for the snorkel goggles to fit the mouthpiece. Oops... rookie snorkelers!

M.J informed us we were unable to snorkel with

NBA and her without the clip. Oh, did I forget to tell you, NBA is also at the Caymans? She was there, and she had been there for a whole week before us, and was having the time of her life.

No snorkeling for us that day, so Mark and I then walked back to Rum Point with no shoes except our floppy snorkel fins. Mark and I decided to wear the fins so that we could walk back on the hot asphalt. Talk about tourist. We looked the part!

LESSON LEARNED
Drinking is needed while in Cayman's!

Kimberly McBee

THANK YOU—for reading to the end.

This is not the end—maybe it's the beginning of another love—writing. I love to tell stories and it's always fascinating to hear the stories that my clients tell. But whatever comes, I know that I'll still be *behind the chair* making people feel and look beautiful.

So... if you are looking for a new look and want to have great results, find a skilled stylist, communicate with her or him. I encourage you to take good professional advice. It's fun to get a fresh image, and in doing so, you are not stuck in the same style from the past.

Embrace change, with your hair, and in most other areas of life!

Last but not least, be kind to your hairstylist—they work harder than you know!

LESSON LEARNED
Happiness is within. *Chair-ish* it!

Made in the USA
Monee, IL
07 September 2021